KW-582-221

'REGIMENTAL PRACTICE'

BY JOHN BUCHANAN, M.D.

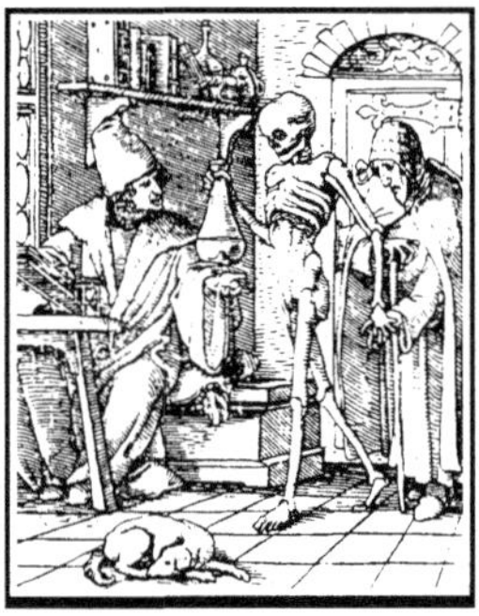

The History of Medicine in Context

Series Editors: Andrew Cunningham and Ole Peter Grell

Department of History and Philosophy of Science
University of Cambridge

Department of History
Open University

Titles in this series include

Anatomical Dissection in Enlightenment England and Beyond
Autopsy, Pathology and Display
Edited by Piers Mitchell

Healing, Performance and Ceremony in the Writings of Three Early Modern Physicians: Hippolytus Guarinonius and the Brothers Felix and Thomas Platter
M.A. Katritzky

The Body Divided:
Human Beings and Human 'Material' in Modern Medical History
Edited by Sarah Ferber and Sally Wilde

Medicine, Government and Public Health in Philip II's Spain:
Shared Interests, Competing Authorities
Michele L. Clouse

Nursing before Nightingale, 1815–1899
Carol Helmstadter and Judith Godden

Secrets and Knowledge in Medicine and Science, 1500–1800
Edited by Elaine Leong and Alisha Rankin

‘Regimental Practice’ by John Buchanan, M.D.

An Eighteenth-Century Medical Diary and Manual

Edited by

PAUL KOPPERMAN
Oregon State University, USA

ASHGATE

© Paul Kopperman 2012

All rights reserved. No part of this publication may be reproduced, stored in a retrieval system or transmitted in any form or by any means, electronic, mechanical, photocopying, recording or otherwise without the prior permission of the publisher.

Paul Kopperman has asserted his right under the Copyright, Designs and Patents Act, 1988, to be identified as the editor of this work.

Published by
Ashgate Publishing Limited
Wey Court East
Union Road
Farnham
Surrey, GU9 7PT
England

Ashgate Publishing Company
110 Cherry Street
Suite 3-1
Burlington
VT 05401-3818
USA

www.ashgate.com

British Library Cataloguing in Publication Data
Buchanan, John.
'Regimental Practice' by John Buchanan, M.D. : an eighteenth-century medical diary and manual. -- (The history of medicine in context)
1. Buchanan, John--Diaries. 2. Great Britain. Army--Medical personnel--Diaries. 3. Great Britain. Army. Royal Regiment of Horse--History--Sources. 4. Medicine, Military--History--18th century--Sources. 5. Austrian Succession, War of, 1740-1748--Medical care--Sources.
I. Title II. Series III. Kopperman, Paul E.
355.3'45'092-dc23

Library of Congress Control Number: 2011944550

ISBN 9780754668770 (hbk)
ISBN 9781409447245 (ebk)

Leabharlann James Hardiman
D2101
Ollscoil na hÉireann, Gaillimh

MIX
Paper from responsible sources
FSC www.fsc.org FSC® C004959

Printed and bound in Great Britain
by Printondemand-worldwide.com

Contents

To my wife, Diane, "a woman of valor"
And our children, Melissa and Aaron ("May you be like")

To my son-in-law, Salif,
And the newest addition to our family, Celina

List of Abbreviations

AL	*Army List*
BHM	*Bulletin of the History of Medicine*
DNB	Dictionary *of National Biography*
Dns.	dragoon regiment
F.	foot regiment
GM	*Gentleman's Magazine*
LM	*London Magazine*
RADCP	Cumberland Papers, Windsor Castle
"RP" Ms.	"Regimental Practice. or A Short History of Diseases common to His Majesties own Royal Regiment of Horse Guards when abroad (Commonly called the Blews)," by John Buchanan [note: this refers to the manuscript version, and will be used to specify page references in that work]
T&P	*Theory and Practice in Eighteenth-Century British Medicine: "Regimental Practice," by John Buchanan, M.D.* [i.e. the extended version of this work, available online]
WO	War Office Records, National Archives

Preface

In 1746, Dr. John Buchanan, recently retired as a medical officer in the British Army, produced a manuscript entitled "Regimental Practice. or A Short History of Diseases common to His Majesties own Royal Regiment of Horse Guards when abroad (Commonly called the Blews)." Revised in several stages almost until the time of Buchanan's death in 1767, this work was for the most part based on the author's observations while surgeon to a cavalry regiment serving in Flanders 1742–45, during the War of the Austrian Succession. When first he wrote it and perhaps for some years afterward, Buchanan may well have planned to publish his manuscript, but in the end he did not. Nevertheless, he left behind a work of great value, which would eventually come into the possession of the Royal Army Medical Corps. It is now included in the holdings of the Wellcome Library for the History and Understanding of Medicine, as RAMC 1037.

"Regimental Practice" is highly unusual in that it is focused on a single British regiment and reflects the perspective of a regimental surgeon. The only other work published in the century that is comparable in this respect is *A View of the Diseases of the Army in Great Britain*, by Thomas Dickson Reide, which reviews the medical history of the 29th and the 60th (3rd battalion) Foot, two units that Reide served successively, mostly in Canada but later in the West Indies, during the years 1777–91. Reide's volume, which was published in 1793, is also of value to the historian. Obviously, however, its focus is on a different war, and a different hemisphere. But perhaps the greatest difference is that Reide's work is deeply colored by his tendency to plead for a therapeutic model that set him rather far from the mainstream in the treatment of many diseases. Buchanan, on the other hand, embodied the mainstream. Reading his manuscript, one sees not only how he treated more than three dozen diseases, as well as various wounds and injuries, but how these conditions were often treated in his time frame.

Buchanan's annotated manuscript will comprise the core of this volume. "Regimental Practice" will be preceded by an introductory chapter that is divided into three sections. The first focuses on Buchanan's life and his career in medicine. The second deals with his medical education, both before and during his years in service, and how personal observation colored his understanding of the cause and cure of disease. Finally, the third section will provide analysis of his practice insofar as it is reflected in the manuscript.

Although Buchanan was almost certainly, as he claimed to be, the recipient of an M.D., and although it is possible that he took some medical courses, whether at university or in one of the lecture programs then available in various major cities, he does not appear to have received much formal education beyond his apprenticeship. Nor is it likely that he was imbued with contemporary medical literature, though he read moderately. In these respects, he was much like many physicians of his time, and like a majority, probably a considerable majority, of surgeons and apothecaries.

Across the decades of the eighteenth century, there were discoveries and fashions that impacted both the theory and the practice of medicine. In the final analysis, however, what is remarkable in the practice of the period is its stability. Various writers of that age, as well as a number of historians since, have conveyed the sense that practice was chaotic. Nevertheless, a review of eighteenth-century medical literature suggests that, on the contrary, the methods used to treat many diseases were fairly standard. It is fair to say that reliance on Peruvian bark to treat ague (intermittent fever, malaria) represented "normative" practice in Buchanan's time, and indeed for the balance of the century and beyond. Mercury for syphilis was also normative, although the amount to be used, the duration of treatment, and the need to promote salivation became subjects of controversy. Diseases that were deemed to be inflammatory were typically treated with large bleedings, while "low" diseases, those whose symptoms suggested a depressed system, were combated by various stimulants and venesection was employed less routinely—by some practitioners, not at all.

When symptoms were poorly defined or appeared to be contradictory, when diagnosis was uncertain, and when initial treatments failed, practitioners often resorted to extemporaneous measures. Treatments for chronic ailments were typically less standardized than they were for acute diseases and the identity of drugs employed in treating given problems varied, not only across the century but within generational cohorts. Nevertheless, the broad rules for treating disease, and even the precise steps for combating certain diseases, were established to the point where the historian may in some cases fairly regard certain tactics as standard and others as eccentric. This is not to argue that the eccentric methods were necessarily unwise—though they often were—or that orthodox therapy was superior, but only that during the century there were methods of treating given diseases that were approved by the consensus and were widely applied. Those who ventured far from them opened themselves to condemnation, especially if their methods failed.

Even within normative practice, however, there was significant leeway. A given disease might generally be treated in part by bloodletting, but how much blood was to be taken, at which stages, and how often could vary significantly in accordance with the predilections and experiences of the practitioner. It is also fair to speak in terms of trends and fashions within British practice. There was a significant tendency toward more moderate therapy after 1750, and this became increasingly dramatic during the last third of the century. For example, a number of writers began to argue that it was not necessary to promote salivation to cure syphilis, and for this reason they came to advocate smaller doses of mercury and a shorter mercurial course than was customary. Nevertheless, the broad message inherent in their therapy—that mercury cured syphilis—was quite standard.

In suggesting that there were norms to practice, I would offer several qualifiers. First, this generalization applies only to those who would have been accepted as "regular" practitioners in the eighteenth century. Quacks did not count among them, even though many had large and elite clienteles. Neither did the various classes of personnel on the medical fringes—purveyors of folk remedies and charms, bonesetters, midwives (aside from the physicians and surgeons who practiced midwifery), and the like—even though this "fringe" comprised the largest group that offered medical or surgical services and often represented the only recourse available to the poor. One might also fairly exclude those that medical professionals dismissed as "country apothecaries." They were seen as ignorant empirics, but what served to disqualify them, like the quacks, was that they were not perceived as entering into, or partaking of, the professional discourse regarding how disease should be understood and treated. Involvement in such discourse was among the distinctive characteristics of the professional practitioner.

A second qualifier is that while the broad strategies for treating disease remained stable, the drugs used in treatment did not. Indeed, drug usage was transformed, to the point where the medicinals that Sydenham relied on were—with some exceptions, notably bark and opium—little used by the late eighteenth century. If one looks for a date to mark the transformation, the strongest case could be made for 1746, when in a new edition of the London pharmacopoeia many traditional simple drugs were unceremoniously cast out and a host of compound remedies were likewise eliminated or were retained only with radically revised recipes. But throughout the century, change was taking place and was being incorporated into professional practice.

History is context. The account of an individual life, the narrative of a battle, the text of a manuscript—none conveys a sense of historical meaning or consequence until it is examined in the circumstance of time and place. The value of Buchanan's manuscript does not lie in the originality of his theory or his practice, but in how well they reflected the norm. Eighteenth-century medical practice was marked by both stability and change, and Buchanan fitted well into this framework.

A Note on the Two Versions of this Work

My book is being published in two versions, one in print and ebook from Ashgate and a second—longer—version that will be made available only electronically. To reduce confusion, the latter version will have a different title: *Theory and Practice in Eighteenth Century British Medicine: "Regimental Practice," by John Buchanan, M.D.* Details for accessing *Theory and Practice* will be available through the author, at p.kopperman@oregonstate.edu.

Both versions of this book include the same preface and introduction, and provide the full text of Buchanan's journal. Nevertheless, there are significant differences. *Theory and Practice* is more than twice the length of the Ashgate volume. Most of the disparity is accounted for by the fact that the annotations of

Buchanan's journal are more numerous and are in many cases quite full; and that *Theory and Practice* includes appendices—particularly two rather lengthy ones, the first on eighteenth-century therapy and the second on the drugs referred to in "Regimental Practice"—that have been omitted from the version that is being published here. Although the additional or extended annotations and the appendices serve various functions, their primary aims are three: to provide as thorough an analysis as possible of Buchanan's practice and the reasoning behind it; to place his practice in context, by comparing it to that of various contemporaries; and to examine trends in therapy across the eighteenth century.

The present version of this work is by far an easier read than is its expanded counterpart. Some readers, however, may choose to consult the fuller version, and fortunately they will have that alternative. In the past, historians were all too often forced to leave much of their best research on the cutting-room floor as they edited their works for publication. Sometimes the paring came at the behest of a publisher. Often, however, it reflected the author's own sense of what might interest the greatest part of his potential audience. The new technology allows for greater leeway, especially for publishers whose desire to produce highly scholarly works is tempered by financial considerations that encourage them to provide for a general as well as a specialized audience. It may well be that heavily annotated primary sources, such as *Theory and Practice*, will within ten years be published only on disks or electronically. This will be hard on those of us who value the tactile relationship to a book in hand, but it should represent an extraordinary boon for researchers and scholars, allowing as it will for access to the full versions of scholarly resources that, owing to cost, can now be published in print only in condensed form, if at all.

Acknowledgments

It is with pleasure, as well as with gratitude, that I acknowledge those who have helped to bring this project to fruition. Sadly, two of those to whom I owe particular thanks are not alive to receive it. The first is Charles Gordon, whom I met in 1986. Charles, a retired businessman, had a profound interest in the medical history of the eighteenth-century British Army, and on learning that I was working in that subject area, he initiated contact. Among the many junctures in our respective research programs was a mutual acquaintance with the Buchanan manuscript, a document that I had first consulted in 1981. Charles had in fact fully transcribed "Regimental Practice," and when we began to correspond he expressed a desire to annotate and publish it, an inclination that I strongly encouraged. By 1989, however, he had abandoned this project in order to focus on producing a doctoral dissertation on Sir John Pringle. It is unfortunate, not only for Charles and his family but for scholars who share an interest in medical history, that he passed away in 1991, before completing his study of Pringle or his still more ambitious work, a history of British Army medical services, 1740–1763. During our all-too-brief acquaintance,

Charles and I exchanged much material that we had encountered in our research, and among other pieces that he provided to me was a copy of his transcription of Buchanan's manuscript. Although my own transcription would differ significantly from his—we took different paths on the issue of whether Buchanan's spelling and punctuation should be modernized—I found his work to be of great use as a point of reference, and it provided me with good leads on primary sources, as well as a head start in translating many of the Latin passages in "Regimental Practice."

A second scholar that I wish to particularly acknowledge is David L. Cowen. Professor Cowen's writings on the history of pharmacy are well known to scholars in that field, and he had a particular interest in British pharmacy. We met at a conference in 1994, and on learning of my interests he kindly provided me with microfilm of more than two dozen books of medicinal recipes from the period 1650–1750, manuscripts that he had examined at the Wellcome some three decades before. This material fits only peripherally into the printed version of the Buchanan journal, but its influence on *Theory and Practice* is significant, since that work includes substantial information on the drugs that Buchanan mentions in "Regimental Practice." Like Charles Gordon, Professor Cowen, who passed away in February 2009, impressed me with his generosity. The eagerness of these two men to enhance my project by sharing the fruits of their research marks the essence of professionalism.

Generosity of a different sort also helped me greatly as I worked to complete this project. In 1998 I was fortunate enough to receive a Burroughs-Wellcome Fellowship, which enabled me to carry out relevant research at the Wellcome Institute. Oregon State University has provided me with two awards through its Research Council, in order to provide stipends for students who undertook tasks related to this enterprise; the OSU Library has granted me several awards to cover the expense of travel in association with research; and the OSU College of Liberal Arts has twice enabled me to purchase release time so that I might pursue my project.

I wish also to acknowledge Patrick Williams, who provided me with extensive notes on the Cowen manuscripts; Dr. Christopher Hilton, who has assisted me in tracking down citations for several manuscripts at the Wellcome Library; and—among the many colleagues of mine who have in some way nudged my project along—two successive chairs of the OSU Department of History, Professors Paul Farber and Jon Katz, who assisted me in obtaining financial support, while also providing constant encouragement.

Other individuals to whom I owe thanks will be mentioned in my footnotes. To those that I have named or will name, as well as to everyone else who assisted me in my work, Thank you.

Introduction

I. John Buchanan and his Manuscript

Sketch of a Life

John Buchanan was born in Drimkill, Kilmarnock, in the Scottish county of Ayr, in February 1710, and was christened there on 22 February. He was the second child and first son of Archibald and Jean Buchanan and was eventually to have six siblings who lived long enough to be christened.[1] In all likelihood, he was the "John Buchannan," son of Archibald, who on 11 January 1729 was apprenticed for five years to an Edinburgh surgeon, William Mcfarland.[2] It may be significant that Buchanan was almost nineteen when he was apprenticed, since it was then more common for boys who were destined for careers as surgeons or apothecaries to enter into apprenticeship between the ages of fourteen and sixteen.[3] Quite possibly medical practice was not the first career option explored by the Buchanans. Financial considerations may also have delayed the move.

On 28 January 1734, a full five years after he was apprenticed, Buchanan was commissioned surgeon to the King's Own (later, "Royal") Horse Guards,

---

[1] The Church of Jesus Christ of Latter-day Saints, International Genealogical Index, Hawaiian Temple Records, batch C11497–2, series #00299–3, pp. 20–22.

[2] P. J. and R. V. Wallis, comps., *Eighteenth Century Medics (subscriptions, licences, apprenticeships)*, 2nd ed. enl. (Newcastle upon Tyne: Project for Historical Biobibliography, 1988), p. 383.

[3] Respecting apothecaries, note Juanita G. L. Burnby, *A Study of the English Apothecary from 1660 to 1760* [*Medical History*, supp. no. 3.] (London: Wellcome Institute for the History of Medicine, 1983), p. 79. My database of 828 men who served in North America or the West Indies as medical officers in the British Army during the period of 1755–1783 (to be appended to my next book, entitled *Lancet and Lance: Medicine, Health, and Sickness in the Eighteenth-Century British Army, with Particular Reference to Army Service in North America and the West Indies, 1755–1783*) yields 16 individuals whose dates of birth or baptism and of apprenticeship can be fixed; for them, the average age at apprenticeship is 15.2 years. In 24 other cases, the birth year, but not the month or date, can be ascertained; if that date is taken to be 30 June, the average for the combined sample (N=40) is 14.9. One boy in the sample was apprenticed at 19, 1 at 18, 2 at 17, 7 at 16, 13 at 15, 11 at 14, 4 at 13, and 1 at 10. One of them was apprenticed to a physician, 29 to surgeons (including 1 barber-surgeon), 2 to surgeon-apothecaries, and 8 to apothecaries.

commonly known as "the Blues."[4] That Buchanan gained the surgeoncy of one of the most prestigious regiments in the British Army when not yet twenty-four should not be taken to indicate that he was seen as exceptionally capable. Rather, the appointment came in association with some house cleaning by the new colonel of the regiment, John Campbell, the second Duke of Argyll. Argyll had also been colonel 1715–17 and during that time he had brought in John Browne as surgeon.[5] When Lord Bolton had become colonel in 1717, he encouraged the surgeon—who, he claimed, was superannuated—to sell out. In established regiments, surgeoncies were normally bought and sold, and within the year Alexander Small, who had served as an army medical officer since 1695, purchased the commission. In a memorial that he later prepared for George II, Small claimed that the transaction price had been "upwards of" £700. He further reported that Argyll, on resuming the colonelcy, had made derogatory comments about him to the King, leading to the loss of his commission "without allowing ... any Consideration for his great Loss."[6] Buchanan now succeeded him. Argyll was probably Buchanan's patron, though the nature and duration of their relationship is undocumented.

In the spring of 1740, Argyll relinquished the colonelcy, and Small put forward the memorial with the stated intention of regaining his commission. Small did not explain in the document why he waited seven years to proceed, but in all probability he held back because he believed that he had no chance for success so long as Argyll was colonel. In a memorial of his own, Bolton corroborated Small's account and supported the petition.[7] Nevertheless, Buchanan retained his place. Small did not obtain another surgeoncy by way of compensation, though it is possible that he received a monetary settlement. Some restitution in terms of cash may in fact have been his aim in petitioning. He was nearly seventy and may

---

[4] William Johnston, comp., *Roll of Commissioned Officers in the Medical Services of the British Army who Served on Full Pay within the Period between the Accession of George II and the Formation of the Royal Army Medical Corps, 20 June 1727 to 23 June 1898, With an Introduction Showing the Historical Evolution of the Corps*, ed. Harry A. L. Howell, repr. in A. Peterkin, William Johnston, and Robert Drew, *Commissioned Officers in the Medical Services of the British Army 1660–1960* [Publications of the Wellcome Historical Medical Library, Historical Monograph Series, no. 14, 1968 (1917)], I, 8 (#148). Johnston refers to him as "Bohannan," the name generally given in the Army Lists.

[5] On Campbell, see the *Dictionary of National Biography* [hereafter, "*DNB*"), his stints as colonel are discussed in (Sir) George Arthur, *The Story of the Household Cavalry* (London: Archibald Constable and Co. Ltd, 1909), I, 354–6. There is an entry for Browne in Alfred Peterkin, comp., *A List of Commissioned Medical Officers of the Army: Charles II to Accession of George II. 1660 to 1727*; repr. in Peterkin, Johnston, and Drew, *Commissioned Officers*, I, 9 (#167), though it does not appear that Peterkin was aware of the break in Browne's service.

[6] On Small, note Peterkin, *List*, in Peterkin, Johnston, and Drew, *Commissioned Officers*, I, 13 (#251). His memorial is in SP 41 (State Papers, Military, 1640–1786), vol. 12.

[7] Small's memorial is undated, but an approximate date can be inferred from the Bolton document (SP 41/12), which is dated 13 June 1740.

have been past it. In any case, he was far beyond the age when most regimental surgeons retired. If he had regained the surgeoncy, he would probably have sold out immediately.

During the first eight years that Buchanan served as regimental surgeon, the Blues remained in England, but in the summer of 1742 the situation changed markedly, as he shipped off with his regiment to Flanders. Since early that spring, British forces had been arriving there. The conflict in which they would participate, the War of the Austrian Succession, had originated in October 1740, on the death of Charles VI, Emperor of Austria and of the Holy Roman Empire. Charles had designated his daughter, Maria Theresa, as his heir, but her accession to the Austrian throne was challenged by the King of Bavaria, Charles Albert. Taking advantage of the turmoil, Frederick II of Prussia invaded Silesia. Soon, various nations were seeking to exploit the weakened position of Austria by appropriating its territories abroad. Of greatest concern in western Europe was the threat by France to seize Flanders. To prevent this, Britain and Hanover, along with the Netherlands and several German states, allied themselves with Austria. The enemy coalition, which included Prussia, Bavaria, Saxony, Sweden, and Savoy, as well as France, appeared to be stronger, but the aims of the partners differed and as a result the coalition failed to pursue a coherent strategy.

During more than three years on the Continent, the Blues participated in a war that even by eighteenth-century standards was slow moving and desultory. The British Army was engaged in only two major battles. On 16 June (27 June n.s.) 1743, it defeated the French at Dettingen, in Bavaria, this victory owing much to enemy blunders. More decisive was the action that took place on 30 April (11 May n.s.) 1745, near Fontenoy, in the south of Flanders. A French army under the command of the French field marshal, Maurice de Saxe, defeated a British and allied force commanded by the Duke of Cumberland. De Saxe followed up his advantage by taking several Flemish cities. He also encouraged a Scottish rising on behalf of the aging son of James II. The spread of this rebellion—the "Forty-Five," as it came to be known—occasioned the recall of almost the entire British force in Flanders. This was largely completed in September and October, and although much of the army returned to the Continent for the final two campaigns of the war, 1747–48, its role was less significant to the allied cause than it had been in the earlier phase. By then the war was winding down in stalemate, and in October 1748 it was concluded by the Treaty of Aix-la-Chapelle.[8]

The Blues were not involved in the campaigns against the Scottish Jacobites nor in the second phase of the War of the Austrian Succession. Although present at Dettingen, the regiment appears to have seen only limited action. At Fontenoy, however, it was heavily engaged and took significant casualties.[9] Perhaps because

---

[8] A good survey of the war is provided by J. W. Fortescue, *A History of the British Army* (London: Macmillan and Co., Ltd, 1910), II, book vii, chs. 4–5, 7.

[9] John Buchanan, "Regimental Practice. or A Short History of Diseases common to His Majesties own Royal Regiment of Horse Guards when abroad (Commonly called the

it was not slated for duty in Scotland, it remained in Flanders for several months after most of the British Army had left, not embarking until 22 February 1746.

Buchanan appears to have been with the regiment throughout its tour abroad and he was present at both of the major battles. In the fall of 1745, however, he made arrangements to leave the service. The commission of his successor, Thomas Cooke, dates from 16 November, but in all probability he did not take up his duties at that time, for it appears that Buchanan remained with the Blues at least until the regiment arrived at Gravesend in March 1746 ["RP" Ms., p. 347; all bracketed page references in the text are to this work, so in subsequent references the source will not be mentioned].[10] Cooke may well have purchased the commission from him. Especially if Buchanan had in the end compensated Small, to whatever extent, it is probable that Cooke reimbursed him, if not more.

After leaving the army Buchanan entered into private practice in Stafford. When the Staffordshire General Infirmary was opened by public subscription in 1765, Buchanan, who had himself donated two guineas, became its first physician.[11] Like physicians at many other hospitals, he received no salary.[12] But the appointment may have benefited his practice and it certainly brought him some kind words, as it did on 15 October 1766, when the general board of the infirmary thanked him and the two surgeons "for their great care and attendance on this Charity."[13] At that point, Buchanan was undoubtedly the most prominent medical man in practice in Stafford and its vicinity.

Buchanan last attended a meeting of the hospital board on 14 January 1767.[14] In early or mid-February he left on a trip, apparently headed for Glasgow. The purpose of his journey is unknown, but in any case he did not reach his intended destination. Instead, he died at Carlisle, on or about 23 February.[15] His death was

Blews)" (hereafter denominated "RP" Ms., with page numbers as in the Buchanan text), the Wellcome Institute for the History of Medicine, RAMC 1037, esp. pp. 155–7, 267–73.

10 On Cooke, see Johnston's *Roll*, I, 17, (#312).

11 The appointment was confirmed by the general board 26 June 1766: Staffordshire Record Office, D685/1/1 ("Records of Stafford General Infirmary – Minute Book of Quarterly General Board, 1765–1820"). Notes of his donation are in D 685/12/1 ("A Report of the State of the Stafford General Infirmary, in the Year 1766") and D 685/23 ("Alphabetical List of Subscribers, 1766–1774, 1824–1825").

12 Neither did the surgeons: Cyril Williams, *The Staffordshire General Infirmary: A History of the Hospital from 1765* ([Stafford:] Mid-Staffordshire General Hospital, 1992), p. 10.

13 Staffs RO, D685/1/1.

14 Staffs RO, D685/2/1 ("Minute Book of Weekly Board Meetings, 1766–1769"), (#42).

15 The brief obituary in *Scots Magazine*, 1767, p. 110, notes the death on 23 February, "At Carlisle, on his way to Glasgow, Dr John Buchanan, brother to the late James Buchanan of Drummikill, Esq; many years a physician at Stafford." *Gentleman's Magazine* reports (p. 144) that death took place on 28 Feb., but in fact the hospital board was informed of Buchanan's death on 27 Feb.: Staffs RO, D685/2/1,(#44).

apparently sudden and unexpected. Buchanan's body was returned to Stafford and was buried there, at St. Mary's Church, on 5 March.[16]

Not quite ten years earlier, on 30 August 1757, he had wed Mary Green at the same church. In the register he is described as a "bachelor" and she as a "spinster," indicating that this was the first marriage for both.[17] If they had children, it is improbable that any survived him. When his widow petitioned the Diocesan Court of Lichfield for letters of administration, she made no mention of children, but she presumably would have had there been any, for such petitions represented an occasion to cite need or distress. The value of Buchanan's estate at the time of his death is difficult to estimate. In submitting her petition, Mary Buchanan, supported by two associates, agreed to put up a £1000 bond to submit a full account of his estate to the court within a year.[18] If the account was submitted, however, it does not appear to be extant. Buchanan himself died intestate, perhaps suggesting that he was in good health as he left for Glasgow in February 1767 and felt that he could afford to postpone the task of preparing a will. The will of Mary Buchanan provides little information on her property or wealth, and it was in any case drawn too late to accurately reflect the estate of her husband at his death.[19]

The Preparation of Buchanan's Manuscript

In all probability, it was shortly after he left the army that Buchanan began work on a manuscript that he entitled "Regimental Practice. or A Short History of Diseases common to His Majesties own Royal Regiment of Horse Guards when abroad (Commonly called the Blews)." The date that he provides on the title page is 1746, and it is likely that he completed the initial draft that year or soon afterwards.[20]

---

[16] Staffs RO, parish register for St Mary's, births and burials 1760–1801.

[17] Staffs RO, parish register for St Mary's, marriages 1754–1787, p. 19.

[18] Her co-executors were Jane Robins of Stafford, who had also been a witness at the wedding; and Joseph Dickenson, the rector of St. Mary's. The grant of administration took place 30 June 1767: Lichfield Record Office, B/C/11. I wish to thank Martin Sanders, area archivist, Lichfield Record Office, for providing me with this citation.

[19] The will of Mary Buchanan, of Johnson Hall, Stafford (PRO, PROB 11/1188/64), was prepared 5 Aug. 1789 and proved the following 27 Feb., by Sir William Winuit, master keeper or commissary of the Prerogative Court of Canterbury. Wills probated at Canterbury often dealt with substantial estates. However, the document provides no insight, specifying only that the entire estate was to be administered and inherited by Mary Buchanan's niece, Mary Meeke, the wife of Rev. Francis Meeke of Johnson Hall.

[20] On p. 201, Buchanan refers to "The Scorbutick Whey of Lond: Dispensary 1747." His reference appears to have been either to the *Pharmacopoeia Londinensis* or to *The Dispensatory of the Royal College of Physicians, London*, by Henry Pemberton, both of which were actually published in 1746. The reference is a later insertion, rather than an item included in the original draft. Given that both works were widely circulated, Buchanan probably used his source in 1747 or 1748, suggesting that the original draft was already completed by then.

"Regimental Practice" appears to have been based on notes that he had taken while in the service. As he states, "it has been my constant custom to keep an exact journal of Regimental Practice" [p. 61]. The manuscript was revised and amended on a number of occasions after 1746, and as late as 1766 Buchanan augmented "Authors on Military Diseases & Gunshot Wounds," a list that he had appended to his journal.[21]

There is a strong possibility that when first Buchanan engaged the manuscript, he was intent on publication. This is indicated by the care he took in revising the original text, correcting misspellings or inserting words to modify statements. It is perhaps noteworthy as well that he was sensitive to the issue of confidentiality. In his manuscript, he conceals the identity of a "Lunatick friend" and refers to soldiers with gonorrhea only by case number [pp. 150, 171].[22] He appears, however, to have abandoned plans to publish. Such is apparent in the notations on the recto (right side, even-numbered) pages of the manuscript, which he left blank as he prepared his initial draft. While in the text written in 1746 he usually includes fairly full and accurate citations for quoted matter, both Classical and contemporary, he often provides just the author's name, and sometimes no provenance whatever, for quotations written on the facing page. It is possible, of course, that he intended to incorporate this new material into a final, polished draft. More likely, however, he at some point decided to forgo publication and rather to continue inserting suitable quotations, sources, and medical observations as they came to his attention.

By 1760, if not before, the War of the Austrian Succession was old news, having been replaced by the Seven Years' War, a conflict of wider scope, more decisive, and far more glorious from a British perspective. Even before this, several publications had dealt extensively with the medical aspect of the Austrian Succession. In 1751, George Cleghorn's highly acclaimed *Observations on the Epidemical Diseases in Minorca* had appeared, and the following year Sir John Pringle, physician to the British hospital in Flanders during the war, had published his landmark study, *Observations on the Diseases of the Army*. Francis Home's *Medical Facts and Experiments*, which appeared in 1759, also dealt in part with medicine during the Austrian Succession.[23] Buchanan may have felt that the medical aspect of the war had been well covered by former colleagues of his and that his own contribution was unnecessary. Furthermore, he practiced in a small city, and unlike physicians in London he had no need to publish in order to enhance his clientele.

---

[21] The latest work listed is Francis Geach, *Medical and Chirurgical Observations on Inflammations of the Eyes. On the Venereal Disease. On Ulcers, and Gunshot Wounds* (Plymouth: B. Law and R. Heydon, 1766).

[22] He is inconsistent, however, in most cases, he does in fact name his patients.

[23] A fourth book also dealt with the medical history of the war, this being James Grainger, Historia febris anomalae Batavae, annorum 1746, 1747, 1748 (Edinburgh: Hamilton, Balfour & Neill, 1753). Perhaps because it was written in Latin, this work does not appear to have been widely read and it was seldom cited in contemporary literature.

II. The Learning Process

Continuing Education

In his memorial of 1740, Small refers to the person who had been given his place as "an Apothecary's Boy from Argyleshire [*sic*] of no education nor competent knowledge." While the characterization was intended to disparage, Small may not have been inaccurate in portraying Buchanan as one whose medical preparation was rather limited. Possibly, Buchanan's education to this point was restricted to what he had learned during his apprenticeship. Nevertheless, his background was no weaker than was that of many men who were newly joined as regimental surgeons and being twenty-four he was at the average age for men who were commissioned surgeons without having first served as mates.[24]

During the eighteenth century, young men who were just entering into practice were not expected to know much—at least, such was the estimate of veteran practitioners. This tolerance extended especially to individuals whose entire training had consisted of an apprenticeship, but also covered those who had in addition attended a lecture course or two. Expectations for young physicians who had completed a university program and received an M.D. were perhaps higher, but not markedly so. At most, men who were early in their practice were expected to be able to correctly diagnose diseases that were quite common and were clearly delineated by symptoms, and to prescribe according to common usage. Confusing or contradictory symptoms might be expected to lead them to diagnose and to treat the disease incorrectly, or to be so uncertain in their diagnosis that they prescribed timidly. Beyond their formal education, medical men were encouraged to improve themselves throughout their careers. Many veteran practitioners would have agreed with the observation of Thomas Fuller, that "physicians, like beer, are best when they are old."[25] Owing to the consensus that men newly embarked in practice

---

[24] Paul E. Kopperman, "The British Army in North America and the West Indies, 1755–1783: A Medical Perspective," War, Medicine and Britain, 1600–1800, ed. Geoffrey Hudson (Amsterdam: Rodopi Press [Clio Medica/Wellcome Historical Institute Series in the History of Medicine], 2007), p. 54. Home's career reflects a common pattern for the period. At first trained by apprenticeship, Home studied medicine at Leiden during lulls in the war. He received his M.D. at Edinburgh in 1750: Edgar Erskine Hume, "Francis Home, M.D. (1719–1813). The Scottish Military Surgeon Who First Described Diphtheria as a Clinical Entity," Bulletin of the History of Medicine (hereafter, "BHM"), 11 (1942), pp. 49, 51.

[25] (Sir) Humphry Rolleston, "Medical Aphorisms, Chiefly in English," BHM, 10 (1941), p. 545. On the stereotype of young practitioners as being easily baffled by complex cases or contradictory symptoms, see John Moore, Medical Sketches: In Two Parts, 1st American ed. (Providence, R. I.: Carter & Wilkinson, 1794), pp. 138–9; and Charles Dunne, The Chirurgical Candidate; or, Reflections on Education: Indispensable to Complete Naval, Military, and Other Surgeons (London: Samuel Highley, 1808), p. 126.

needed extra guidance, a considerable body of medical works was generated to assist "young and unexperienced practitioners."[26]

The military was looked on as a place where young practitioners could hone their skills and acquire knowledge through observation and study. That such service provided good training in surgery was a belief of long standing, as reflected in the Hippocratic adage, "If you wish to be a surgeon, follow the army."[27] But if army service proved useful to the surgeon, it was of even greater value to the individual who hoped to practice medicine on returning to the civilian world. For young men trained as surgeons or apothecaries, the army experience represented an opportunity to study medicine. Despite his title, the regimental surgeon's practice was generally more medical in nature than surgical.[28] Even a few years of service would afford him the opportunity totreat a considerable range of diseases, as well as injuries.

Many experienced medical men also saw advantage in army service, as they enjoyed an opportunity to observe the manifestations of disease and the success of treatments on a large scale, and thereby to test theories that they had learned or developed. While serving in Flanders, Pringle wrote to his friend Andrew Mitchell, "the <love of the> Study of my Art encreases daily. I have double pleasure now in reading Medical books, because I can turn theory into practice, confirm from experience my former Speculations or at least be sure they have not been just."[29]

As a physician, Pringle had impeccable credentials, having pursued medicine at Edinburgh, then moved on to Leiden, where he studied under Herman Boerhaave—"the teacher of all Europe," as Albrecht von Haller called him. After receiving his M.D. at Leiden in 1730 he returned to Edinburgh, where he was soon appointed a professor of metaphysics. By the outbreak of the war, he already had a significant reputation in the medical profession.[30] Few of the men who served as

---

[26] The quotation is from John Ball, The Modern Practice of Physic: or a Method of judiciously Treating the Several Disorders incident to the Human Body (London, 1760), I, ii.

[27] This advice is derived from an observation by Hippocrates in "Physician" (du médecin), c.14.

[28] Reide reported, "Surgery forms a very small part of a regimental surgeon's duty, except in an active war": A View of the Diseases of the Army in Great Britain, America, the West Indies, and on Board of King's Ships and Transports, from the Beginning of the Late War to the Present Time (London: J. Johnson, 1793), p. 284. Richard Brocklesby noted the statement of a former regimental surgeon who had served in several hard campaigns: "in full seven years, he had never met with near 100 properly chirurgical cases in the whole regiment; though in that course of time, near 2000 men had gone through the regimental books": Oeconomical and Medical Observations, In Two Parts, From the Year 1758 to the Year 1763, inclusive. Tending to The Improvement of Military Hospitals, and to The Cure of Camp Diseases incident to Soldiers (London: T. Becket and P. A. De Hondt, 1764), p. 48.

[29] Ghent, 31 Feb. 1743, BL, Add. 6861, f. 188.

[30] The DNB provides a brief sketch of Pringle's career. A fuller review of his early career, through the peace of 1748, is included in Dorothea Waley Singer, "Sir John Pringle

medical officers in the British Army during the War of the Austrian Succession had received an education comparable to his, but many of them may have undertaken medical studies beyond what an apprenticeship would have afforded. And a significant number studied medicine in a formal program while they were in the service.

During his time in Flanders, or more likely after he left the army, Buchanan wrote a response to an assertion by the German physician, Johann Degner, that regimental surgeons were ignorant, illiterate, and generally no better than quacks:

> Our Regimtal Surgeons from the beginning are generally well educated; wheither they are to profess Physick or Surgery have the same education, first serving an apprenticeship are instructed in all the particular branches of medecine & Surgery by proper Professors, attending the Lectures two or three years; & for further improvement travele to forreing [*sic*] universities & attend hospitals, of wch Paris & Leyden have been the most remarkable; some go to Montpellier making the tour of Italy, afterwards many take to the army in order to pass some years, & there officiate as Physician, Surgeon & Apothecary; tho young Practitioners are sure of practice & may improve by experience; supposing equal capacities the advantage most [*sic*] be very considerable. [Degner fragment[31]]

Possibly in this statement Buchanan in part describes himself. Perhaps he had enrolled in a few medical courses at Edinburgh while still serving out his apprenticeship to Mcfarland. It is also possible that he attended medical lectures in London during the years 1734–42, when his regiment remained in England, or that he did so in Brussels or elsewhere after it moved to Flanders. If attendance at lectures required that he be absent from duty, he probably reserved this study for the four to six months each year when the Blues were in winter quarters, for the workload would have been light and other surgeons could have handled it.

With greater certainty, it can be said that Buchanan learned from other medical officers and shared information and ideas with them. It appears that Home, who was then a regimental surgeon, accepted Buchanan's account of an autopsy [*RP*, n. 48]. By the same token, Buchanan accepted the observations and conclusions of Adam Austine, another regimental surgeon, in the wake of an autopsy that the latter performed [p. 64]. And Buchanan and these contacts were further associated in a network whose cohesiveness and value may well have been unexcelled in the contemporary civilian world.

> I'm intimately acquainted with the greatest part of the Regimental Surgeons of our Army ... We have a weekly Club w<h>ere all are welcome to come, the chief Subject of conversation relates to our own business; it being a standing rule with us, that if any thing remarkable happen'd during the last weeks practice, it's to

---

and His Circle," Annals of Science, 6 (1949), pp. 128–33.

[31] The "Degner fragment" appears at the close of "RP" Ms.

> be made publick for the good of the Society; by this means we know the practice of the whole army during the Campn, & in winter quarters that of the Garrison, where we have an opportunity of attending the hospital. All talk freely, nor can I perceive any reservedness or fondness for Secret medecines, or a private method of practice; some are regular bred Physicians. [Degner fragment]

Not only were regimental medical officers in regular contact with their peers, but they also interacted with senior personnel who in general far outdistanced them in terms of education and experience. This contact was not always welcome. During Buchanan's time in Flanders, and indeed throughout the Austrian Succession and the Forty-Five, medical services in the field were dominated by Pringle. Imperious and often impatient, he freely imposed his authority on regimental medical officers, and a series of commanders-in-chief enforced his directives. In the wake of Culloden, the battle that broke the back of the Forty-Five, Cumberland ordered: "Dr Pringle recomends to the Regtal Surgeons timous bleeding in the feverish & Pleuritick disorders, if for the future such patients are sent to the Hospitals without bleeding complaint will be made of the Surgeons."[32] But while Pringle was often headstrong in promoting ideas that he regarded as being established truths, he believed passionately in sharing information and analysis with peers in his profession. In February 1743 he wrote to Mitchell of the progress that he was making in his study of "Garrison Diseases," the project that would grow into his greatest work. He reported,

> By the advice of Genl. Ligonier I am to write to the Director of the French Hospitals for an account of their diseases, & at the same time promising them toutes nos Lumières & he does not doubt of their Correspondence. I mentioned the thing to Ld. S[tair]. who was of the same opinion. I propose by the same advice & authority to demand of the proto Medicus at Vienna a History of the Austrian Garison & Camp diseases, which will not only satisfy my curiosity in this way but be of service to ourselves when exposed to the same hardships.[33]

It was not just the elite of the profession that Pringle sought to engage. Over the years, he would build a trans-European network of correspondents, one of the largest circles that centered on any British physician of his century. It not only included major figures like von Haller, but also a number of medical men who were distinguished only by the fact that, for some reason, they had gained his respect. Buchanan himself was included in the circle, at least early in the Austrian

---

[32] National Army Museum, acc. #6807–228–2 (Cumberland's orderly book, 7 Dec. 1745–26 June 1747), order issued at Inverness, 22 April 1746.

[33] Aix-la-Chapelle, 2 Feb. 1743 n.s., BL, Add. 6861, f. 190. In France there was, by royal authority, a program of medical correspondence among the military hospitals, and the practical observations that were collected were supposed to be made public. Medical Commentaries, 2 (1774), p. 152.

Succession. According to him, when in 1743 an epidemic of pleurisy struck "all over Europe ... Dr. Pringle [who] was then at Aix la Chapelle with Lord Stair, wrote a short account of it in that place, begging the same from me" [pp. 113, 115].

Medical service in the military provided a foothold for the practitioner who returned to the civilian world. Medical service in the military was accepted by government as a significant credential, for men who had practiced surgery in the army and navy were permitted to practice as surgeons or apothecaries without obtaining the license of the Company of Surgeons. This privilege was first given governmental sanction during the Cromwellian period, but more important was a statute enacted in 1749. The company made several attempts to enforce its monopoly over practice, but failed. An act in 1815, which imposed penalties on unlicenced practitioners, was largely undone by a second act, which, in 1825, permitted former military surgeons to practice as apothecaries without obtaining license. Only in 1858 was the exemption removed.[34]

On the title page of "Regimental Practice," the author styles himself "John Buchanan M.D." The question remains, however: When and where had he received his degree? In all probability, it was at a university that did not require attendance. The most likely candidates would have been Aberdeen and St. Andrews. Neither had a medical program during the eighteenth century, yet both granted M.D.s to many individuals, including a significant number of active or former army medical officers. Aberdeen may be slightly the more probable of the two, in that it bestowed more degrees and the chancellor of Marischal was Archibald Campbell, who on the death of Buchanan's mentor in 1743 succeeded him as the third Duke of Argyle.[35] The published records of Aberdeen and of St. Andrews do not list Buchanan as a recipient of an M.D.[36] Nevertheless, it is likely that he received the degree from one of these universities, probably in 1746, just after he left "the Blues", and that the relevant record is either not extant or has not been located. It is, on the other hand, highly improbable that he merely styled himself an M.D. without obtaining the degree. In eighteenth-century Britain it was not unusual to address

[34] Lloyd G. Stevenson, "A Note on the Relation of Military Service to Licensing in the History of British Surgery," BHM, 27 (1953), pp. 420–27, passim.

[35] DNB.

[36] I have consulted i.a. the following works, none of which contains a reference to the granting of a diploma to an individual who may have been Buchanan: List of the Graduates in Medicine in the University of Edinburgh from MDCCV to MDCCCLXVI (Edinburgh: Neill, 1867); W. Innes Addison, comp., A Roll of the Graduates of the University of Glasgow: From 31st Dec, 1727 To 31st Dec 1897 (Glasgow: MacLehose, 1898); Peter John Anderson, comp., Fasti Academiae Mariscallanae Aberdonensis: Selections from the Records of the Marischal College and University MDXCIII-MDCCCLX (Aberdeen: New Spalding Club, 1898); R. W. Innes Smith, English-Speaking Students of Medicine at the University of Leyden (Edinburgh: Oliver and Boyd, 1932). I wish to thank Paul Farber for having reviewed Innes Smith's extensive manuscript list of medical degrees granted in the 18th century by various European Universities. Also, my thanks go to Michelle Gait, for her report on the relevant records at King's College, University of Aberdeen.

a regular medical practitioner as "doctor," regardless of his credentials.[37] Even quacks appropriated the title. But for a practitioner to set out as a physician and claim that he had an M.D. when such was not the case was a very different matter. If the imposture were discovered, his practice would be ruined. The community of physicians in Britain was small and elite, and in consequence the likelihood of exposure was high. Furthermore, it was fairly simple and inexpensive for an experienced practitioner to acquire the degree. In September 1746 John Hawkins, who like Buchanan had served the British Army in Flanders, noted in his journal:

> at the Marshall College in Aberdeen I had a Diploma for Doctor of Physick granted me, I having first had Certifycates of my being Qualifyed of Dr. Char: Alston Professor of Botany at Edinburgh, and of Dr. Pringle our Physitian to the Army, as also from Dr. James Gordon Principal of the Colledge at Aberdeen who also gave me his fees which was 5 pounds for our being intimately acquainted while I lived at Aberdeen, the remaining fee was ten pounds, which I paid to an Agent at Edinburgh upon receipt the Diploma, which was sent after me ther.[38]

Someone with Buchanan's record could easily have taken the same route to a diploma, and this makes it all the more improbable that he laid claim to an M.D. that was not his. Buchanan himself recognized and accepted the significance of credentials in the medical hierarchy. In his original draft of "Regimental Practice," he refers to a regimental surgeon, Adam Austine, as "Mr." At some later point, Buchanan changed the title to "Dr." Very likely this came after Austine received an M.D., in 1749 [p. 64, n. 45].

Certainly Buchanan's contemporaries and peers accepted him as John Buchanan, M.D., and his career as a civilian practitioner was in part dependent on this. By the mid-eighteenth century, a physician—though not an apothecary or surgeon-apothecary, who might also practice medicine—was expected to have the credential. That for two decades Buchanan practiced as a physician in Stafford and that he was appointed to serve as the first physician of the Staffordshire General Infirmary are tacit evidence that his community regarded him as having an M.D. Almost certainly, such was the case.

---

[37] With some exaggeration, William Stevenson wrote that "all practitioners from farriers to physicians" were called doctors: Considerations on the Dangerous Effects of Promiscuous Blood-letting (Newark, 1783), p. 40. Thomas Champney suggested that physicians, surgeons, and man-midwives alike might be styled "Doctors of Health": Medical and Chirurgical Reform Proposed, from a Review of the Healing Art, throughout Europe, particularly Great Britain (London: J. Johnson [etc.], 1797), p. 84. It might be noted that Champney was himself a surgeon and midwife and as such may have coveted an elevated title.

[38] Wellcome Library for the History of Medicine, WMS 2788 (Journal of John Hawkins), f. 23r.

In appears that Buchanan was disdainful of ignorant practitioners. As has been noted, he challenged Degner's condemnation of regimental surgeons, but only in that the latter applied it with a broad brush, implicitly taking in the British. He did not disagree when Degner's characterization was directed elsewhere:

> he is very severe on all Quacks, to them he joins Camp-Surgeons, saying their Education is at first in the barbar's Shop, then learning to bleed & dress slight wounds, & from being attendants at chirurgical operations, become profess'd Surgeons & are appointed as such to some troop or Company, where they practice at ... random & learn a particular method. afterwards assume the name of Doctors[.] this may probably be true in his Country, & is customary in Germany & the Low Countries, all Barbars practising Surgery, commonly illiterate, tho some are smatterers in Latin, entirely ignorant of Anatomy, few or none having ever seen a Desection, nor is the profession much esteem'd. they have hardly a book, nor do they knowe any. [Degner fragment]

Buchanan likewise condemned the bonesetters of his own country. Especially galling to him was that they, like other fringe practitioners, enjoyed a fair degree of credibility: "Im perswaded many Sprains pass for Dislocations amongst the English Bonesetters, & that they put in my [*sic*] bones which were never out. apply their infallible Searcloth, & obtaine great reputation by the person walking abroad in a few days" [p. 215].

When Buchanan entered the army, he may not have been much more than the "apothecary's boy" dismissed by Small. By the time he left in 1746 however, he was in all likelihood far better schooled in practical medicine than were most practitioners of his age. His involvement with the army network played a significant part in this development. He probably benefited as well from the medical literature that he read during his time in service. Here, however, the evidence is less consistent.

Sources

One can only guess which books, or how many, Buchanan had available to him during his service on the Continent. His personal collection was probably small, perhaps being limited to what he could take with him on the march. In addition, Buchanan may well have shared books with colleagues, especially when the army was in winter quarters. Years later, Robert Hamilton, a former medical officer, complained, "It is unfortunate for the soldiery, that the regimental surgeons must apply in general so little to books."[39] As has been noted, Buchanan began his

39 Robert Hamilton, The Duties of a Regimental Surgeon Considered: With Observations on His General Qualifications; And Hints relative to a More Respectable Practice, and Better Regulation of that Department (London, J. Johnson [etc.], 1787), I, 340.

journal in 1746, after he returned to civilian life and presumably had more books at his disposal.

The manuscript as first composed is heavily geared to Classical sources, the number of references suggesting that Buchanan already had a good grounding in this literature. Hippocrates is, by far, the medical source that he refers to most often in "Regimental Practice," as he quotes him no fewer than 77 times (and cites him once), drawing on thirteen works.[40] Moreover, 53 of the references come in the 1746 draft, the remainder being later interpolations. Although possible, it is improbable that he first examined the Hippocratic corpus in 1746, even as he was preparing his manuscript. The remaining Classical authorities on medicine and science pale by comparison. Celsus he quotes only four times, on each occasion briefly, and none in the 1746 version. The remaining sources in this category are all noted in the original draft, but are of little consequence in Buchanan's manuscript. Pliny is quoted twice—the same passage—and Dioscorides is cited once. Perhaps most significant, Galen is mentioned only once, and even this is a secondary reference [p. 99]. Possibly Buchanan knew of Galen only from references that he had read or heard. His lack of first-hand knowledge and, apparently, of interest reflect the low estate of Galenic influence in eighteenth-century British medicine.

Buchanan's use of Hippocrates far transcends what convention would have called for. It was common for medical writers of his time to quote ancient authorities in the course of their works, whether these references were meaningful in context or were merely inserted to display erudition. Generally, however, the quotations were brief, aphoristic, and few in number. Buchanan, on the other hand, quotes frequently and often at length. His tendency is so exceptional that there are few if any parallels in eighteenth-century British publications that are focused on contemporary medicine.

In his 1746 draft, Buchanan also makes extensive use of non-medical Classics. Easily his main sources are Ovid (65 references) and Horace (64). In all, he utilizes works in this category 180 times, 121 in the 1746 draft, and only once in the form of a citation, rather than a quotation.[41] Quotations from the Classics serve as the primary medium for him to display emotion. His own diction suggests detachment and dispassion, while Classical passages convey humor, irony, excitement, and pathos.

Buchanan appears to have enjoyed a genuine facility in Latin. Several of the books of Hippocrates were available in English translation, yet when he quotes from them he does so in Latin, almost certainly from the popular translation of the complete works that the French physician, Anuce Foës, had first published in 1595. Buchanan could likewise have made use of English translations of a number of Roman literary figures, Ovid and Horace among them, yet he chose to quote

[40] The data on Hippocrates, and on all sources, is tabularized in app. A, T&P (note: the appendices are available only in this online version.)

[41] The cited source is Xenophon ("RP" Ms., p. 334), coincidentally the only Greek in this category (though Buchanan presumably knew his work in translation).

in Latin. Among modern European languages, he may have known French, but perhaps not fluently. It is noteworthy that as regards most French works that had been translated by the time Buchanan wrote—Charles Rollin's *Roman History*, Montesquieu's *Reflections on the Roman Empire*, Montaigne's *Essays*, Samuel Tissot's *Essay on Bilious Fevers*—he cites or quotes only the English version. He does cite the French titles of *L'eloge l'yvresse* and of Bernardini Ramazzini's *L'art de conserver la santé des princes* (ironically, a translation from Latin), but he quotes neither.

Buchanan's evident fluency in Latin and knowledge of Roman literature raises significant questions regarding his education, but unfortunately it does not answer them. He probably had not enjoyed a Classical education in the exalted sense that the term carried in the eighteenth century, but somewhere along the way he had received a good grounding in Latin and an introduction to at least the most prominent Roman writers. By contrast to the more than 200 references to Classical authors in "Regimental Practice," more recent literary figures are mentioned seldom. George Buchanan is cited twice—for that matter, works in Latin—and John Buchanan quotes Charles Aleyn and James Thomson once each. He cites or quotes from another fifteen sources on non-medical subjects, but just two (*L'eloge de l'yvrsse* and Rollin) are referred to in the 1746 draft. Only three of the remaining thirteen, however, were published before 1746.[42] And the total number of references to works in this category is only about half that given to either Horace or Ovid alone. Still, it does appear that after he left the service Buchanan began to expand his acquaintance with modern literature, as well as with the Classics.

Despite Buchanan's reverence for Hippocrates, his manuscript not surprisingly reveals some knowledge of post-Classical literature on medicine. He does not cite any medieval or Arab works in his text, nor does he mention any Renaissance authority. Among post-1550 writers, Friedrich Hoffmann receives the most citations—fifteen—but he is never quoted. Notable by his absence is Boerhaave.[43] In the 1746 draft, Buchanan cites or quotes only four modern writers: Ramazzini, Ysbrand van Diemerbroeck, David Abercromby, and Nicolaas Tulp. Five additional references to Ramazzini were inserted later, suggesting that Buchanan continued to consult his work. Although an edition of Hoffmann's complete medical works was available as early as 1740, Buchanan cites it only in interpolations made after 1746. Of sixteen sources added after Buchanan completed his original manuscript,

---

42 These three are Verulam (Bacon)—in an apparent misascription—Pereira, and Montaigne. Journal of the Campaign on the Coast of France, 1758 and Biographia Britannica were both published after 1746, as were the works by the following: Carte, Cooper, West, Smollett, Leland, Salmon, and Secondat (Montesquieu). Parker was published in 1746.

43 Buchanan does note that the recipe for a preservative medicine against gout "is said to be originally from Dr. Boerhaave" ("RP" Ms., p. 159), but he does not cite or quote any work by him.

seven were published before 1746, but these may not have come to his attention until afterwards.[44]

Buchanan refers to only one modern work on surgery, that being John Ranby's influential *Treatise on Gunshot Wounds*. He quotes Hippocrates at length on surgical matters, notably dislocations and fractures, and he cites Lorenz Heister's *Medical, Chirurgical, and Anatomical Cases and Observations*, but only in a medical context. The list of Buchanan's references does, however, suggest that he was keeping up with advances in medicine. Most of the modern works listed are post-1700, and eight were published after 1750.

The significance of which works that Buchanan refers to in the draft as completed in 1746, rather than in later interpolations, is considerable. For the most part, "Regimental Practice" is about the methods that Buchanan used to treat diseases and injuries encountered in the Blues 1742–45. Sources that he quotes or cites in the original draft may conceivably have helped to shape his method. Of course, one should not assume that the works that he refers to represented the full range of his relevant book learning at the time. They may simply have been the ones closest to hand or, if he sought a quotation, the most quotable. Nor is it certain that Buchanan himself read every work that he cites, or even that he quotes. It is quite possible, for example, that at least two of the three quotations that he provides from Giorgio Baglivi's *De praxi medica* were drawn from an English treatise (not published until 1758) in which they are likewise quoted ["RP" Ms., nn. 51, 322]. Despite these qualifications, it is worth bearing in mind which of the sources that Buchanan refers to appear to have been known to him during his service in Flanders.

As has been noted, Buchanan concludes the manuscript with a list of books on military medicine and surgery. While relevant to the theme of his journal, Buchanan's list is rather remote from the broader work. Only one publication included in it, Ranby's treatise on gunshot wounds, is referred to in the text of "Regimental Practice."[45] Buchanan was probably familiar with some items on the list, like Pringle's *Observations on the Diseases of the Army*. But in all probability, he consulted only a few, and most items on the list were just titles to him. Many of them were quite obscure, including dissertations written more than a century before. Moreover, several were in languages that Buchanan apparently did not know, as evidenced by his notations (*Germaniae*; *Belgiae*). Most of the older studies mentioned in the list would have been little known by his contemporaries, while ironically Buchanan fails to include a single work by Ambroise Paré,

---

[44] These include the works by Hoffmann, Baglivi, Castro, Piso, Degner, Weber, and Turner. Sources published after 1746 include Tissot, Whytt, Young, Russell, Degner, Johnstone, Heister (the work that Buchanan cites), and Huxham (vol. I of Observationes). Although the ed. of Pharmacopoeia Londinensis that Buchanan cites was published in 1746, he puts the date at 1747, and he probably did not in fact encounter it prior to that year.

[45] Buchanan lists a treatise by Hoffman; however, he does not refer to this piece itself in the text.

arguably the best known and most influential of all military surgeons. The eclectic and somewhat eccentric nature of the list suggests that Buchanan copied it from one or more that he found in print. Unlike the rest of his journal, which clearly was revised and amended a number of times over the course of perhaps two decades, this list may have been prepared all at once, since the hand is rather regular and only one work, Donald Monro's study of diseases treated in army hospitals 1761–63, appears to have been squeezed in. Buchanan left room for additions, however, and it is noteworthy that all works on the list that were published after 1746 appear at or near the end of their alphabetical grouping. It is probable, though not certain, that Buchanan prepared the list not long after he completed the first draft of his journal, then embellished it as additional works came to his attention or were published. The list is in essence a coda, neither feeding into nor drawing from Buchanan's text. Still, the fact that he went to the trouble of preparing it suggests, as does other evidence, that as of 1746 and probably for several years beyond he had it in mind to publish "Regimental Practice."

Insights that Buchanan picked up through reading undoubtedly helped to shape his therapy and his general understanding of medical issues. But the manuscript suggests that he did not pattern his practice on any particular authority. He cites Hippocrates extensively and he accepted some broad precepts that were common to both Hippocratic and eighteenth-century medicine. Nevertheless, the methods that he used to treat specific diseases were often quite different from those advocated by the master. For example, Hippocrates recommended treating gout with external applications, while for his part Buchanan apparently advocated dietary means to moderate the disease and also used bloodletting and purgation [p. 165]. Buchanan also questions the value of "critical days"—the belief that fevers reached their crises according to a set pattern—although it was one of the hallmarks of Hippocratic medicine [p. 99]. Indeed, while he may have quoted Hippocrates more than did contemporaries, he followed him less than did many. Hippocrates appears to have been merely a point of reference to him. The same can be said of his other sources. They encouraged speculation on his part, and they may have influenced the way in which he treated diseases with which he was not familiar. But there was no authority that he followed slavishly.

Learning Through Observation

Significantly more important than books in Buchanan's learning process was observation. He readily applied in his practice insights that he had drawn from his own observations or from those of colleagues. Likewise, he was quick to challenge conjecture that went against the evidence. This evidence he searched for in several ways.

One was through autopsies. The postmortem of a dropsy victim, apparently not performed by him, caused him to note, "no water in the thorax, contrary to expectation, for some imagined he had been suffocated by water in the breast" [p. 155]. The ready availability of cadavers for dissection represented one of the greatest advantages that medical officers in the military held over civilian practitioners. In a letter that he wrote to his mother in May 1809 William Dent, who was tending soldiers at Colchester, commented, "I am very glad that I came here for besides attending the sick and wounded we have the privilege of dissecting those who die and in London we could not get a dead body under three Guineas."[46] Buchanan discusses fourteen postmortems in "Regimental Practice," additionally noting that a number of victims of dysentery were dissected during an epidemic in 1745 [pp. 64, 65, 67, 69, 71, 129, 131, 139, 141, 142, 153, 155, 293, 331]. Since he generally discusses the operations in the passive voice, the agent is often unclear. However, Buchanan's use of the first person establishes that at least two of the postmortems were conducted by him and that he observed a third, while several were clearly conducted by others, the results simply being reported to him. Clearly, postmortems were common if not routine, and they provided Buchanan—and, in all probability, many of his colleagues—with a significant learning tool.

Buchanan also observed surgical techniques, and he appears to have been quite willing to adjust his ideas on therapy in accordance with what seemed to be working. Assessing in his journal the use of setons to treat consumptive patients in the hospital, he observes, "I suspected these Seatons would produce carious ribs, which never happened, for they always worked outwards towards the skine." Better yet, "these Seatons discharge largely & I have seen some recover to admiration, were formerly walking Skeletons now fat & plump & free from Cough" [p. 167]. In another instance he comments, "I have imagined Buboes might be opened by Caustic befor they were quite ripe, & that the discharge after the Eschar cast off would be sufficient, & by this method shorten the cure, not waiting for Suppuration; but then the Gland remains undestroyed, having never suppurated; is hard, proves tedeous work to the Surgn & great pain to the patient" [p. 183].

When he attempted to divine the origins and potential treatments for diseases, Buchanan, like many of his contemporaries, compared groups that were confronted by the same disease but contracted it in sharply different proportions. Frequently the groups were distinguished by status. Troopers were somewhat better clothed and accoutered than were foot-soldiers, and this Buchanan saw as having an impact on health. In his journal, he writes of ague, "the foot more subject to it than the horse, being more exposed to the injuries of the weather in doing Duty, having no watch-cloaks. our Troopers have a good warm cloake & strong boots, & less duty" [p. 33].

---

[46] Leonard Woodford, "A Medical Student's Career in the Early Nineteenth Century," Medical History, 14 (1970), p. 92. Hamilton complained that while autopsies were an excellent learning tool for young regimental surgeons, they seldom performed them. He noted that the disposal of bodies was under the control of the officer commanding the regiment, but that he was usually quite willing to permit dissection: Duties of a Regimental Surgeon Considered, I, 213–14.

Buchanan regularly observed differences in the prevalence of epidemic diseases between officers on the one hand and their men on the other. In "Regimental Practice," he notes the disparities, but does not always seek to explain them. So, for example, he reports that in the Blues only men, and not officers or their servants, contracted the disease that he calls "yellow fever" in 1742, but he does not speculate on the significance of this [p. 61]. Like virtually all contemporaries, he recognized gout to be primarily a disease of the elite or, in the context of the army, the officers [p. 161]. More often, however, he observed that diseases afflicted the troops more than the officers. Of the itch, which raged among the rank and file during the crossing to France in 1742, he notes, "None of the Officers had it, and only two of their servants, as they dayly attended their Masters, were obliged to keep themselves clean, the Disease might be prevented" [p. 15]. Observing that officers and their servants were likewise free of the flux and griping that struck many men in the Blues during the spring of 1743, he cites a number of distinctions that made them less liable: "being less exposed to the injuries of the weather, have good dyet good wine. wine and water for their common drink, good lodgings, good fire, [and] are warmer cloathed than the men" [p. 25].[47]

The pattern in which a disease struck might cause Buchanan to explain its cause a certain way while rejecting alternative possibilities. Of an outbreak of ague in 1742, he observes, "None of the Officers have been ill of this desease, nor any of their Servants; a plain proof that the air of this Country is not the only cause of the distemper, but that it rather proceeds from the Soldiers manner of life. few of the inhabitants were ill of this" [pp. 35, 37].

Buchanan was willing to allow contrary evidence to overthrow his theories. When pleuretic fevers struck in 1743, he and Pringle exchanged notes on the disease and framed their respective theories to account for it. Pringle, who was in Aix-la-Chapelle,

> had himself for a Patient & blamed at first the sunk Situation & Sulphurous air. I imagined it was greatly promoted amongst our men from their being quartered in publick houses, the Beer much better than at Ghent, cheap & good measure, & they indulg'd pretty freely, sitting much by the Stoves, we had pleasent Sunshine weather, yet the air was cold, mornings frosty & winds N:E: the Officers dress more & change cloaths oftner than in last quarters & therefor more subject to catch cold, the ramparts are very pleasant & evening walks were frequent.

But having noted some problems with each attempt to link the disease to particular circumstances, Buchanan recognized the ultimate difficulty: "had it not appeared Epidemical & universal, both Dr Pringle & I would have remained satisfied with our own private theory" [pp. 115, 117].

---

[47] Ibid., p. 25. Buchanan also reported [p. 24] that spring recruits did not contract the disease, for they joined the Blues when the weather was warm and dry.

The way Buchanan weighed evidence to determine the cause of disease is well illustrated by his comments on a dysentery outbreak that afflicted the army in 1742.

> Some say it proceeds from eating fruite; & others from catching cold on Duty. the Distemper decreased as the fruite went out of Season, though the drinking of beer continued. The latter end of September & beginning of October were remarkably wet and cold, which no doubt promoted the distemper & I believe was the chief cause, especially as we came from a better quarters to a worse, and doing night Duty to which we were strangers at home. The Streets here [Bruges] are very flat, & when the raine falls it lyes long, which makes the Streets wet. tho not dirty the feet are always wet and damp: nor are the Flemish Shoes so good as the English ... None of the Officers were ill of this distemper and only three of their Servants, being less exposed to the injuries of the weather, have good dyet good wine. wine and water for their common drink, good lodgings, good fire ... are warmer cloathed than the men; plenty of ripe fruits of which they eat freely, nor do they seem to be unwholesome. [pp. 23, 25]

In this passage and elsewhere, Buchanan dismisses the traditional belief that dysentery was caused by eating fruit [cf. pp. 287, 288, 291, 309]. Here, and indeed in most controversies on the cause of disease, Buchanan stands with the consensus of contemporary British authorities, rather than the older view.

In "Regimental Practice," Buchanan often cites popular belief regarding cause or cure of a particular illness, then judges it by his own observations. In some cases, he seems to credit legend: "Some are frighted at the sight of a person lately recovered, & imagine themselves to be infected; go home with this notion, are uneasie & sicken, having complaints the same as preceeding the eruption, & should be treated in the same manner as if the pocks were at hand. & tho they do not appear at this time, & the person recover, I have seen them come soon thereafter" [p. 57]. Generally, however, his impression of the evidence leads Buchanan to doubt tradition. On the basis of his observations, he discounts what he claims to be a common belief: that apoplectics are carried off by the third attack [p. 328]. Elsewhere, he writes, "It is a common notion that a sudden fright will cure the ague. January 14th 1743 Ashberry of Major Jenkinson's troop was almost recovered of an Ague & that day sent a foraging, fell into the *Scheld* unexpectedly, was heartily ducked and frightened; yet the Ague returned at its usuale time more violent than formerly, & was afterwards cured by the Bark. the same happened to our Sutlers Servant, but instead of curing the Ague, occasioned a violent inflammatory fever" [pp. 27, 29].

In a number of instances noted in the journal, Buchanan's own observations cause him to question popular ideas on causation: "others imagine [smallpox] may be caught from change of air. viz: going from one place to another, yet I never observed any thing remarkable of this" [p. 57]. He challenges the contemporary tendency to explain the prevalence of particular diseases in terms of a national constitution, observing that "Scorbuticke complaints are not so frequent as one would expect, as they are said to be predominant in every English constitution" [p. 197]. Nor does he fall in line with the widespread belief that each nation was characterized by different physical attributes: "it's commonly said that a wound on an Englishman's leg is not easely cured, but I don't think them as bad as reported, tho many are Subject to swelled legs being full of humours" [p. 207]. Sometimes he discounted interpretations that he had heard or read, and substituted his own, as in this observation: "Swelled testicles are frequent, & said to be occasioned from astringent medecines & the Surgeon always blamed; but are rather from catching cold, riding, intemperate drinking & private debauches, & are very obstinate in old venereal constitutions" [p. 177].

Buchanan's nosology was not very rigorous. In reference to a "camp fever" that struck in 1743, he rejects assertions that the disease was new, supporting his argument only by quoting a report that Sir John Spelman's death in 1644 was caused by "the camp-disease" [p. 298]. The tendency to identify different diseases with each other, and then to interpret their nature and determine treatment on this basis, was characteristic of the period. It helped to bridge the gap between empirical and rational medicine.

III. Buchanan's Practice

The Military Circumstance

While there was a broad coherence to medical practice in eighteenth-century Britain, there was also variation that in part accorded with the practitioner's circumstances. A physician who practiced in London and enjoyed a wealthy clientele would have dealt with his patients differently and prescribed differently than would have a small-town apothecary whose clients were poor or lower middle class. Buchanan's circumstance during the years 1742–45 was the army. The scope of his practice, the health problems that he dealt with, and his relationship with his patients were greatly influenced by this.

In passing, "Regimental Practice" reveals many aspects of army life, including the rigors of the march, the violence of battle, and the tedium of winter quarters. Readers even learn that Buchanan for a time kept a young fox as a pet and that many troopers became fond of it. Nevertheless, the journal is not a desultory discourse on life in the Blues. References to the march, battle, and camp mainly provide background to explain disease or injury. The fox is introduced so that Buchanan can make a point about the impact of diet on behavior [p. 94].[48]

[48] Buchanan also notes (ibid., p. 221) the case of a puppy that lived at his lodgings. Again, however, the reference is in a medical context i.e. that when the puppy's thigh bone was broken it healed without bandaging or being immobilized.

Buchanan occasionally places himself in the military context. Of the days before Dettingen he recalls, "we talked so much of decamping every day, that for Six nights I did not put off my cloaths, nor boots, lay on the ground & happy if I could get a little straw in a Soldiers tent" [p. 263]. But recollections of his own experiences are few. Even when Buchanan recounts his bout of ague in 1743, he presents it as a case history [pp. 39, 41]. He often writes in the first person, but usually just to give his opinion or recount his practice regarding some medical matter. "Regimental Practice" is emphatically not about Buchanan. Nevertheless, much about him can be inferred, especially as regards his relationship with the men and officers of the Blues.

Characteristically, in his manuscript Buchanan never indicates a motive for having entered the military. He appears, however, to have been attracted to the army life and mission. The term of his service was exceptionally long for a regimental surgeon, and he chose to accompany the Blues on foreign service, rather than sell his surgeoncy before the men embarked, as did so many colleagues when they were confronted by service abroad. Given the number of his quotations from martial literature and the focus of his literary and historical sources, ancient and modern, it appears that Buchanan had an interest in Roman military history and more generally in the romance of warfare. His coverage of action that he himself had seen is, however, very slight. He recalls Dettingen with some appreciation of the carnage it brought: "its impossible to describe the variety of wounds from Cannon Shot, small arms, swords & Bayonets" [p. 267]. However much felt, however, such observations are so few and brief as to appear perfunctory. Rather than communicate in his own words, Buchanan strings quotations to evoke the horror of warfare, while focusing his commentary on such matters as how the wounds of battle were treated.

Unlike Pringle, whose position and authority were largely dependent on the whim of the high command, Buchanan does not appear to have been much caught up in army politics. He seems to have admired Lord Stair, Pringle's primary patron, and he lavishes praise on his performance and leadership at Dettingen [pp. 265, 267, 268]. But he does not even mention the officer who succeeded Stair as commander-in-chief, Field Marshal George Wade, and he makes note of Cumberland, Wade's successor, only in reference to a wound that the Duke received at Fontenoy [pp. 269, 322].

As a regimental surgeon, Buchanan's primary responsibility would have been to the 250–300 men and officers of the Blues, though he would also have been expected to tend their wives and children, as well as farriers and laborers who served the regiment. The level of difficulty faced by army medical officers varied markedly, according to the situation. When the army was in winter quarters, their duties were generally light, but they might be inundated in the circumstance of battle or epidemic. Buchanan himself could be overwhelmed by the flow of patients. Of a flux-like illness that struck the Blues in 1743, he writes, "by the midle of Augst it was so common that I could not keep a list of the mens names or cases" [p. 281]. In some respects, however, Buchanan's responsibilities were heavier than was usual in the army. Occasionally, perhaps regularly, the Blues appear to have suffered from a shortage of nurses. This shortage may well have forced Buchanan to assume a heavier burden and probably had a negative impact on the quality of care, as he himself observes in regard to patients suffering from inflammatory fever: "Many complaine of not being well nursed; when they have an appetite, & victuals not ready at that time, the appetite is lost again; as we have no regular nurses the sick are nursed by their Comrades, & it cannot be expected that they are so carefull in giving their medecines, as they ought to be" [p. 97]. Men who had their wives with them were better nursed. Buchanan notes that the troopers' wives "often apply a warm ... Dishcloath to the Throat, & sometimes a hot loafe" in the event of their husbands' suffering an attack of quinsy [pp. 123, 125]. However, either because they were unmarried or because their wives did not accompany the regiment to Flanders, only a small minority of men enjoyed this advantage in nursing. Furthermore, as in other horse regiments, Buchanan had no mate, which presented difficulty in times of crisis. He recalls that in the wake of Dettingen, "having no assistant [I] avoided amputations as much as possible" [p. 267].

In an epidemic, the workload of medical officers increased not only because of a spike in the number of patients, but also because of a reduction in the number of nurses that they could call on. During an outbreak of flux and fever in 1743, reports Buchanan, "the Nurses dyed so fast that private Soldiers were obliged to nurse their Comrades" [p. 283]. Like many medical officers, Buchanan valued nurses who were capable and conscientious. Of an epidemic of bloody flux in 1744, he observes, "We had many private receipts as infallible, but I would rather trust good nursing than family medecines" [p. 289].

To reduce his workload, Buchanan could have utilized the general hospital extensively. The hospital was intended to handle chronic cases or diseases that were regarded as dangerous and likely to be protracted. It typically provided separate wards or facilities for patients who were suffering from contagious diseases. Invasive surgery was typically performed by hospital, rather than by regimental, personnel, though in emergencies, as were common in the wake of battle, regimental surgeons handled many amputations. Buchanan himself appears to have sent out the more serious surgical cases. He may have been reluctant to perform lithotomies [p. 142].[49] He reports in his manuscript that while in the Blues simple fractures were treated in barracks, "Compound fractures being more difficult of cure & requiring much time are sent to the Hospital" [p. 223]. On the whole, however, he appears to have been reluctant to send men to the hospital, for he perceived a number of dangers.

> Surgeons should not send triffling cases to an hospital: those who go for slight Surgery cases are in great danger of catching some distemper of the house viz. fever, small pox &c. Harris of Cpt. Shipman's having dislocated his collar bone

[49] This case occurred when he was in civilian practice.

> attended with great contusion was sent to Tournay hospital; got a slowe fever with great variety of complaints, took a dislike to the house from seeing so many disagreeable objects, continued in a lingring way some months, was at last brought to his Barracks at Brussels, tho we had a good Hospital there, would not be perswaded to go to it, but chose to die in his qtrs always thinking of what he had seen in the hospital. Some are naturally lazy & indolent & are much more so after being some time in the hospital. [p. 196]

As is reflected in this quotation, Buchanan, like many contemporaries, was concerned that the military hospitals bred epidemics. In his view, the wards were too large and so encouraged contagion [p. 321]. A hospital base being quickly set up in the face of crisis was likely to be especially unhealthful. Buchanan writes of one facility that was established soon after the engagement at Dettingen.

> Here our hospital was in great disorder as their baggage was not yet arrived from Flanders, the Sick lyeing on straw only in Barns, Stables, outhouses, &c: there was commonly a Dunghill befor the Door where all their Pots, Bedpans, &c: were emptied, & stinke abominably in warm weather, & great swarms of vermine are dayly produced; those Dunghills are lower situated than the Street, & when raine falls the common Channel empties … itself into the Dunghills, carrying much filth along with it, & after raine the stench was almost insufferable. [pp. 281, 283]

Buchanan's anecdote regarding "Harris of Cpt. Shipmans'" also speaks to the concern that men who were confined long in hospital facilities often fell victim to depression [cf. p. 295]. When the Blues were due to depart for England, troopers who remained in hospital became profoundly depressed at the prospect of being left behind. According to Buchanan, "When the mind is so greatly concerned, the body is soon affected, grows restless & unease, tossing & tumbling in bed, nor have medecines the same effect … whether given internally or applyed externally, nor do wounds suppurate so kindly in this condition … three dyed last night unexpectedly, all being greatly concerned at the thoughts of being left behind, & telling their Comrades they should certainly dye. all earnestly wished to return home, yet many dyed" [pp. 339. 341; cf. p. 343].

Yet another concern expressed by Buchanan and others was that transportation to hospital caused great physical and mental stress. Not only were hospital facilities sometimes far off, but during the winter some facilities closed, and hospitalized patients were routinely transported many miles to bases near headquarters, with consequences of the sort noted by Buchanan in reference to an evacuation in late 1743: "the Sick were brought down the Rhine in Barges; suffered much from cold & wet & bad provisions, were Sick, faint & weake, pains in all their bones, Limbs numb & threatning a mortification" [p. 258].

In the wake of Dettingen, Buchanan visited the hospitals of the French, the Hanoverians, and the Dutch, and compared their practice in treating wounds. He has little to say about the Dutch in his journal, other than that they followed a rather rigid, though simple, method of dressing wounds and that their preference when in garrison was to place their men in civilian hospitals. He is, however, quite critical of French practice: "French … Surgeons went round the hospital carrying a tub of Brandy & Syringes, with which they washed the wounds, dressing with dry lint dipt in brandy, & covering with digestive. Such of their wounded as could be transported & require time to recover, were sent to the nearest French towns. the wounded lay on Strawe or hay in houses, churches, Barns &c: our men say the French bleed often & cut much." Of the three facilites that he observed he appears to have been the most impressed by that of George II's duchy.

> The Hanoverians had their hospital baggage in the field; their hospital was soon put in good order; their men in good houses, lye on palliases stuffed with Straw, have good coverings; their dressings are very neat of drawn lint, wounds cleaned with fine Spunge, soaked in warm water & brandy, use the caustic on the first appearance of proud flesh … hospital medecines are carried on a large waggon, divided into many different partitions, & opening at many places; any particular medicine may be easely got at, the whole easely packed & unpacked … use many chemical preparations. [p. 284]

Buchanan's endorsement of the policy and practice of the Hanoverian ally, and his deprecation of those of the French enemy, may have reflected bias, but a number of eighteenth-century British sources—objectively or not—echoed the observation of his informants that "the French bleed often & cut much."[50]

Buchanan accepted that some hospital facilities were of high quality—as was noted above, he did write of "a good Hospital" at Brussels—but for many reasons he preferred the infirmary even to the best of them. He favored a facility that was small, uncrowded, and well-aired. In his manuscript he notes that during a smallpox epidemic in 1743, "two Troopers were seized with this distemper in Camp, & removed to the neighbouring village, were distinct & favorable, lay in an open barn & had a slight flux during the whole course of the Desease" [p. 51]. On this count, too, he would have rejected the hospital when possible, preferring instead that the men be treated in the infirmary, the type of facility where he practiced.

Buchanan's Relationship with his Patients

Like a number of other writers on military medicine, Buchanan stresses the importance of treating acute diseases quickly. Of pleurisy, he writes, "one day's delay may cost the patient's life" [p. 109; cf. p. 103]. However, soldiers were

[50] Paul E. Kopperman, "The Drive toward More Moderate Therapies in British Medicine, 1750–1800." Proceedings of the 37th International Congress on the History of Medicine (2002), pp. 267, 270n3.

notoriously reluctant to visit the infirmary. Even less willing were they to be confined in a hospital facility. According to Buchanan, one victim of a camp fever that struck in 1743 "would neither eat nor drink, nor taste medecines, saying he was certaine he must dye, & did dye in his tent. our men had taken a dislike to the hospital, would rather suffer the injuries of the weather in the field, or think themselves happy if they got into a Boners out-house & lye on straw" [p. 295].

The first inclination of sick or injured soldiers was to treat themselves, as did the men who attempted to cure itch (scabies) with burnt gin [p. 19]. Buchanan reports that when soldiers, on leaving their ships, scraped their shins on the ropes, they rubbed brandy on the wounds [p. 7]. While not in this case commenting on the wisdom of their practice, elsewhere in his manuscript Buchanan does express concern over the tendency of the men to doctor themselves. As regards chilblains, for example, he observes, "the men rub with ol: tereb: as soon as they perceive them. tho looked upon as triffles yet are frequently of dangerous consequence & ought not to be neglected" [pp. 225, 227]. Similarly, Buchanan notes that soldiers from Essex used groundsell to control ague fits, and that he tried it, but did not find it to be effective [p. 37]. He also reports that men and officers treated themselves for scurvy [pp. 199, 201]. And line officers on occasion took it upon themselves to treat their men, sometimes unwisely. Buchanan records the case of a lieutenant in the Blues who misinterpreted the stitch of one of his troopers as a sprain and applied a cerecloth, nearly bringing about the death of the patient [p. 213].

Often medical officers were hampered by a code of masculinity that encouraged soldiers to play down their problems. Even in the face of serious diseases or conditions, the men often responded with bravado: "Peerage, of Col. Beakes's had it [phimosis] to a great degree & would not suffer anything to be done, being a Farrier only rubbed with Ungt. Dealth. & continued so two years, laughing that he now got a natural scabbard, & swearing he would never draw his sword. was lately discharged" [p. 175].

Buchanan depicts the trooper as a difficult patient. He was, first of all, partial to rigorous treatments: "Troopers love to be worked heartely, & so much the better if it operates upwards & downwards, & seldom blame a strong vomite but will always find fault with a weake one" [p. 77; cf. p. 173]. Buchanan's patients were often demanding and self-centered. He writes, "Soldiers often grumble at seeing nought but dry Lint & old rags applyed to a wound ... & think themselves neglected if they are not dressed once in 24 hours whether necessary or not" [p. 268]. Troopers were prone to be contemptuous of treatments and medicines that struck them as being too simple or commonplace. When Buchanan advised fever patients that they could relieve headache by bathing their feet at night, they at first ridiculed the practice as "a childish thing," only to adopt it when they observed it working [p. 89]. For coughs, Buchanan recommended licorice, but recognized that it had a fault: "that of being too common, & therefor by some despised" [p. 107; cf. p. 127]. There was a similar problem in the case of jalap, which he regarded as an excellent vomit, yet disparaged by the vulgar "from being cheap & so much in practice" [p. 173]. Buchanan used mercurial pills of his own design to treat venereal eruptions and found them to be effective, but "our men only found fault with them as being so small and having no violent operation, imagining medecines can have no good effect unless they be rough in their operation" [p. 187]. And while Buchanan criticized his patients for disdaining remedies that were too gentle, his manuscript suggests a broader problem: that they were often reluctant to take the drugs that he prescribed. For example, according to him, the men had a "foolish aversion" to theriac, an opiate, as a remedy for tenesmus [p. 282].

In other respects, too, the men were prone to be uncooperative. Buchanan complains, "it's a difficult task to cure the private man of claps: when the painfull Symptoms abate, they neglect taking medecines, let the running continue till it turns to a Gleat, then say they were not well cured. Officers are more easely cured & that with the very same medecines, being more carefull of health & keeping a proper Regimen" [p. 171]. He later adds, "Venereal emptions on the Skin are common amongst us, & I have been often afraid to attempt a cure without Salivating from the difficulty represented by Practical authors, but our men have neither time nor Patience for this method" [p. 185]. In a number of instances, Buchanan points up the unwillingness of soldiers to cooperate in prolonged treatment. He reports the case of a trooper who fractured his ischium, then insisted on getting out of bed and walking before it healed. He was therefore left lame, with one leg shorter than the other, and was in consequence recommended to Chelsea [p. 219].

If men were reluctant to seek medical treatment, there was perhaps still greater cause for them to reject surgery. Various factors, however, allowed many to endure it. Shock, pain, or apprehension might cause patients to faint on the operating table [p. 279]. And just as men who were drunk were prone to injury, so might their drunkenness reduce the pain of corrective surgery [p. 219]. Even patients with no palliative, however, might endure surgery with fortitude. According to Buchanan,

> Majr. Jonston of the horse Guards received a Cannon shot on the left anckle, the bones smashed to pieces & the foot hanging by the great tendon, the large arterie bleeding at … full stream. I stiched the artery, cut off the anckle, dressing dry with proper bandage &c: leaving the amputation of the leg to a more convenient opportunity. it's surprising how some people bear pain better than others, this Gentleman never changed his voice or altered his Countenance; when I told him You must loose your leg, he answered cooly, that shall be the work of another day. [pp. 267, 269]

But not all patients were stoical in the face of pain. They often resisted treatments that might prove painful. After observing that an accidental evacuation of blood cured chordee, Buchanan speculates that the condition might be relieved by venesection, but adds that no one would allow him to apply a leech to the affected region [p.175]. The men also had their vanity. According to Buchanan, when their parotids swelled during colds, they feared that if they suppurated it would leave scars [p. 124].

Buchanan reports in his manuscript that some men with buboes "complaine of so much pain as not suffer You to touch it. are even afraid if You look at it" [p. 181]. Symptoms that medical men knew not to be worrisome might nevertheless terrify their patients. So, for example, the troops who were suffering from dysentery might be alarmed by the loss of even a little blood [p. 289]. Buchanan appears to have accepted his patients' fears and, to the extent possible, taken them into account in determining therapy. A common device of his was deception. In the course of his discussion of inflammatory fever, he observes, "Some people have a certain prejudice against vomites … I then order them to drink two or three quarts warm water in order to wash the Stomach, &often provides a good emetick: let the patient be never so sick, he is easely perswaded to drink warm water when freightened at the name of a vomite" [pp. 73, 75]. Of another condition he notes, "A Blister applied to the part often removes the Stich; & when applyed without forewarning the patient there are no great complaints; but if You mention a blister, he will plead an excuse, saying he is yet not so bad & beg to put it off till tomorrow. if You tell him of a plaister to the part he is well pleased & applies it with pleasure, nor are his complaints troublesome" [pp. 107, 109].[51] Buchanan also withheld information when he thought that this benefited the patient. On one occasion, a cornet broke his collar bone. Buchanan set and bandaged it, without telling his patient of the break, and the bone quickly healed. "Had he been informed of this fracture," he observes in his journal, "he would surely be blooded, gone to bed & keeped his Chamber some days" [pp. 221, 223].

Buchanan complains that soldiers tended to blame doctors for not curing them, even when they were responsible, as by discontinuing their therapy once they appeared to be on the mend: "I would rather undertake the cure of Bubo than that of a Clap. so long as they require dressing the men attend dayly for fear of being poxed, & never pretend to cure themselves; but their private receipts for claps are infinite. when the cure is compleated they don't mind physick or any regimen, but return to the old way, & if poxed thereafter blame their Surgeon" [p. 183]. If venereal patients were a problem, so were those with ulcers on the leg: "tho they appear to the eye a meer triefle yet they are always tedeous & sometimes never cured. a Surgeon gets no credite by them; the men will not keep a proper Regimen; You can hardly perswade them to take a Dose or two physick, the good effect of which is soon overballanced by the nixt debauch … The men ride or walk dayly … despising such small sores, & find fault with their Surgn for not curing them" [pp. 201, 203, 205].

Despite Buchanan's reservations about his patients, when sick troopers came to see him, he tended to trust their judgment. He regularly asked them what they

---

51 Hamilton reported, "I have on many occasions seen an apparently strong and robust man tremble at the sight of a lancet, and faint away in the course of the operation, who, I dare say, would have undoubtedly charged the enemy with fixed bayonet, or mounted a breach without fear. There is something abhorrent in our nature at the deliberately wounding our flesh." Duties of a Regimental Surgeon Considered, I, 255.

believed had made them ill and sometimes drew plans for treatment from their interpretation of cause. In one instance, he notes that a number of troopers were suffering gripes after bouts of flux: "Upon asking what occasioned this Distemper, I was told by some, they believed it proceeded from drinking white Beer, I advised them to abstain from Beer & drink small milk punch" [p. 21]. On another occasion he interviewed patients suffering from rheumatic fever and learned that "all blamed cold as the first cause" [p. 121]. Sometimes the men could not give a plausible explanation, leaving Buchanan to speculate, as in the case when "three men were ill [of jaundice] in one roome, for which they could not give any particular reason, having messed with their comrades. probably from too gross feeding & little exercise; the men are apt to indulge too much on coming into garrison" [p. 133].[52] He also questioned patients about the progress of their treatment, as in the case of fever sufferers that he treated for nausea: "The morning after the vomite they often find themselves much better, being more *lightsome* as they express it. I then enquire into the state of their body, whether they go to stool or if their belly feel full, which if it does, purging is necessary" [p. 79].

Buchanan had a keen interest in folk remedies that the troops employed, and he reports on many of these in "Regimental Practice." He notes, for example, that there were different remedies for ague tried by Irish recruits and by troopers from Essex [p. 37] and observes, "there are many private receipts for the cure of an Ague, and every body has his own favorite, & I have been complimented with many, & it would be endless to mention them ... upon recovery some of the men eat a Lemon with its skin on such days as they expect the fit" [pp. 29, 31]. In most cases, Buchanan does not evaluate these remedies. In some, he approves. In the course of discussing sudorifics for fever patients, he notes, "The men deal much in hot pots for this purpose; or treacle posset, boyled beer or buttered ale; & no <bad> medecines if they are not made too strong" [p. 85]. Nevertheless, he does criticize some of the remedies that the men applied to themselves. In respect to the itch, he comments, "some men cure themselves with Mercuriale water, Viz: boyling two pennyworth Corrosive mercury in a quart spring water into a pint, and washing the parts affected. This is too corrosive and often excoriates the parts, & sometimes raises blisters, striking the itch suddenly inwards, whence proceed violent coughs and diseases of the breast" [p. 17].

Buchanan appears to have been willing to tailor treatment to the comforts of his patients. Of smallpox sufferers, he writes, "Acid Sharp drinks are longed for <about> the latter end of the Desease & may drink freely of small Sherbet, adding a little wine so to be a pleasant cordiale" [p. 47]. To some extent, the issue at hand was in fact the comfort of the sick. "Drought is a constant attendant of fevers & very troublesom to the Patient ... Acid sharp drinks are often wished for, & I know none so pleasant as the common sherbet made rich with fruite, of this the sick seldome tyres, tho he soon dislikes all other drinks" [p. 81]. But of course food and drink played an important part in therapy, as well, and often illness affected

[52] More on importance of exercising, p. 135.

appetite. In the case of fever patients, Buchanan reports, "I often consult the appetite & seldom forbid what the Patient wishes for, unless it be something very much out of the way" [p. 91].

The preferences of Buchanan's patients influenced the therapy that he provided. On at least one occasion, Buchanan bled at the request of a patient [p. 295]. The attitude of his patients in any case encouraged bloodletting: "on every slight fall or bruise the trooper thinks himself neglected if he is not blooded" [p. 209]. And it was not only patients who pressured him in respect to therapy. Officers sometimes complained that he was not treating their men properly. A captain in the Blues wondered why he was unable to cure a man's cold [p. 127]. Several officers were angry when they learned that men in their units had not been bled, although they were suffering from fever, this being a form of fever that did not, in Buchanan's opinion, respond well to venesection [p. 295].[53]

Buchanan tried to protect patients from being ordered to duty by their superiors or pressured into it by other soldiers: "their Comrades think nothing of a broken shin, saying they have had as much at foot ball & cured it with a leafe of tobacco; grudge doing duty for their lame Comrade & often oblige him to do his Duty befor he is well. but in order to save him <I give> a certificate *unfit for Duty a horse back* directed to his Officer" [p. 207].

While Buchanan may on occasion have come into conflict with officers over how best to treat his patients, he shared their concern that many men simply feigned illness in order to avoid duty. Suspecting that some venereal patients magnified complaints of nocturnal pains, only to be exposed as frauds [p. 191], he sanctioned deception to expose them:

> Some pretend to be sick or Lame & uncapable of Duty but can do some work in the hospital when employed as servants, & have good wages. these are not easely detected, tho sometimes discovered by making them drunk, & carefully observing their motions. a Stiff Knee is a common complaint, but upon being fudled, can dance, jump, & cut capars ... Some suffer the part to be blistered, Seatons cut &c: but have recovered upon hearing the Surgeons whisper that a red hot iron must be applied for nine mornings in order to remove that humor from the bone. [p. 196]

Buchanan took a hard line again malingerers, but he accepted that some soldiers genuinely believed that they were ill, even when in fact they were not. He appears generally to have sympathized with these men, and he again approved of deceiving them, in this case to provide them with peace of mind: "We have many imaginary Venereals, & when one of a Troop is fluxed for venereale complaints, if any of his old Companions have the least aching pain in their bones from catching

---

[53] In the same regard, Hamilton complained of "the murmurs of officers, if men are not so soon cured of their complaints as their anxiety would have them": Duties of a Regimental Surgeon Considered, I, 58.

cold or scabs on their skin from itch or scurvy, presently reflecting on their past life, conclude themselves poxed & are not satisfied without fluxing" [p. 193; cf. p. 195].

Like many writers on military medicine, Buchanan saw depression to be a major problem in his regiment, and in his journal he expresses sympathy with the sufferers. "Soldiers sometimes take a melancholy turn, become lowe spirited, senseless & childish, avoid company, cry or mutter to themselves, love to be solitary. upon asking their case, they tell long stories about their past & present condition, are in great fear of being some way or other lost" [pp. 327, 329]. Even soldiers who were recuperating from a slow fever in 1743 remained "greatly low-Spirited, & despairing of doing well, & fearing being left behind. which is always the case with Soldiers & greatly prevents recovery, their Mind being never easie" [p. 295]. Buchanan observes that soldiers—by inference, heavy drinkers—who suddenly swore off strong liquor were especially prone to melancholy, while a "heartie bottle" offered at least short-term relief to the problem [p. 329].

Accounting for Disease

At a number of points in "Regimental Practice," Buchanan notes the opinions of officers and men regarding how they contracted their diseases. It appears that in most cases he credits this conjecture, and in no instance does he absolutely reject it. So for example he reports that a man who contracted yellow fever "thought his illness was occasioned by the fatigue of marching" [p. 62]. Two officers who died of a slow fever in 1743 had, he notes, regularly slept on the ground, on straw alone, and both had complained of catching cold at the outset of the disease [p. 297].

Buchanan generally accepted contemporary wisdom regarding etiology. He saw obstructed perspiration as a frequent cause of disease. It might be the cause in itself or the trigger to a chain reaction: "the [yellow fever] patients commonly complained of catching cold on Duty, perspiration seemed to be obstructed and to have fallen on the bowels" [p. 63]. He also held to the common belief that ague was caused by wet ground or unclean air and conversely that dry weather or a cleansing of the air, as by snow, would reduce the danger [p. 43].

The nature of contagion interested him, as it did many of his contemporaries. The itch was one of the diseases that he considered contagious. "This disease is never to be rooted out, one man affects a whole barrack in winter Garrison and his tent Mates in the summer. Some are cured sooner than others, and he who is last acuring gives it fresh to his Comrades" [pp. 15, 17]. But he also recognized the principle of natural immunity: "I blooded many Itchy Troopers, yet never catched the distemper. & I know a *Scotch:* Gentlemen who was never affected with it, though he has had many an itchy bedfellow" [p. 19]. In a similar vein, he wrote, "Some constitutions not easely affected with the small pocks" [p. 55; cf. p. 56]. Of acquired immunity, however, he was less certain, for the evidence seemed inconsistent: "it's no extraordinary thing to have [smallpox] twice or thrice, & I have been assured of the same from their Physicians. Mr. Stevenson, Surgeon to Durure's Regimt assured me he attended on one of his Soldiers twice for this distemper since he came to Ghent" [p. 45].

The bond between disease and heredity likewise appears to have interested Buchanan, for he refers to a possible linkage in several instances in "Regimental Practice." Of the plethora that occasionally afflicted a major in the Blues he comments, "this is a family distemper" [p. 100]. But he also looked for alternative explanations for diseases that appeared to run in families. He notes the case of a father and his son (a trooper in the Blues) who were prone to colic, but observes that both drank large quantities of milk, meaning that diet, rather than heredity, might be responsible for their problem [p. 237].

Nevertheless, to Buchanan's mind, the main cause of disease was the weather. Like many eighteenth-century medical men, he studied the weather in association with patterns of health and disease. In 1744, he wrote, "During this Campn I keep't an exact journal of the weather from a small Thermometer, as to heat or cold, wet or dry; and accordingly observed my return of Sick & Lame, rise & fall like a weather Glas" [p. 313].

Overwhelmingly, Buchanan cites as causes factors that were associated with exposure and were as such intrinsic to the life of a soldier, particularly a soldier on the march. Mentioned most often are cold and chill; rain or dampness; stoppage of perspiration; and fatigue. Singly or in combination, Buchanan specifies these as causes in no fewer than 57 instances. A sense of the linkage that he detected is provided in his report of an epidemic of bloody flux that beset the army in the wake of Fontenoy: "it was not universal, being confined to such troops only, as had most fatigue. alarms were so frequent amongst our out parties, that there was scarce time to pitch tents, or untye cloaks, all lay on the cold ground exposed to the open air, & tho the days were warm the nights were cold" [p. 291]. In accounting for disease, Buchanan often paired overheating with a subsequent stoppage of perspiration, typically being the result of an overheated man becoming chilled.

Avoiding Disease

In some cases, Buchanan resisted explanations that blamed the soldiers for their diseases. Of an outbreak of blood flux in May 1745, he notes that the troops' consumption of fruit could not be used as an explanation, since fruit was not yet in season, "yet irregularity must be charged to the poor Soldier & gin is blamed; yet I have always observed the drunken Soldier the most healthie, but when seized with Sickness, often attended with greatest danger" [p. 291]. Nevertheless, he believed that the army leadership, and even the soldiers themselves, could do much to maintain health.

That officers and men faced particular danger when their units engaged is obvious, and in "Regimental Practice" Buchanan discusses the wounds and injuries that resulted from combat. The fact that the Blues were involved in only two battles, however, and were deeply committed in only one, during their three-plus years on the Continent suggests that the hazards of battle did not generally affect the health of the regiment. Nevertheless, even when there was no combat, military life was often fatiguing and stressful. The British did not see significant action in 1744, yet the proximity of the French caused hardship.

> About the latter end of Augst. our Duty began to be very hard and fatiguing from out parties, forraging, &c: the covering party for forraging turning out at break of day, & the forragers an hour or two thereafter. worke hard all day in cutting corn, mowing Grass, making trusses &c: and don't return till evening; the old Grand Guard is often employed on this duty, are thirty or forty hours a horsebacke, & often without forrage. we sometimes went fifteen miles in search of forrage, (which at home would be reckoned a long march) & return with heavie trusses, the men mounted. Some parties were ordered out over night, in order to cover the forragers nixt day, were obliged to lye on their arms in the open field, stand to their arms all nixt day, & return to Camp at night & often wet to the skine, & some accidents of Gunshot wounds from skirmishing with the Enemies out parties. [pp. 309, 311]

Nor was the impact of battle on the health of the army to be measured only in terms of wounds and injuries. Troops suffered greatly from overheating and fatigue, and Buchanan blamed these for an epidemic of fever that struck after Fontenoy [p. 322].

Buchanan often laid the health problems of soldiers to the military circumstance. As he saw it, costiveness was often the result of poor diet [p. 3]. Walking and riding in boots caused legs to swell [p. 249]. And as was noted earlier, the group of causes that he cited easily the most often were particularly associated with the exposure to the elements that was inevitable when the army marched.

The troops certainly suffered from exposure when marching, but their living conditions in camp and garrison were likewise inimical to health. Even while in winter quarters, they often lived in damp quarters [p. 13]. Tents became worn out during the campaign, so that by fall they were insufficient to guard the men from cold and damp [p. 305]. And in summer heat, they presented another danger, according to Buchanan: "one can scarcely believe how desagreably hot a <Soldiers> tent is on a warm day. I have much adoe to bear it whilst I ask a sicke man how he does, being almost ready to faint. they are changeable from heat to cold to a surprizing degree, the perspiration sometimes greatly promoted and then suddenly checked" [p. 257].

While much of the sickness and injury suffered by the troops was intrinsic to life in the army—the fatigue and exposure associated with marching, the occasional battle—the men also harmed themselves by engaging in certain behavior freely. The vigorous lifestyle that characterized the army sometimes led to injury. Buchanan reports that the men often suffered head bruises when they fell while learning to iceskate [p. 211]. A cornet in the Blues dislocated a finger as he attempted to catch a cricket ball [p. 217]. The military ethos as it related to costume could also impact on health. According to Buchanan, the faces of officers became sunburnt as the Blues rode through Germany in 1743, but they would not shield themselves by uncocking their hats, for this they considered "unmilitary" [p. 251].

Buchanan's formula for maintaining health was quite standard: "Spare dyet with good exercise & light wines seems to be the best preservative from Distempers" [p. 311]. He stressed the importance of regularity and advocated a diet that included toast soaked in oil and oily broths, along with exercise, for individuals who were sometimes costive or who followed a studious or sedentary life [p. 143].

The circumstances in which the soldier functioned might promote health as well as illness. Even when men were on the march, moderate, dry weather served to maintain them. Comparing the health of the troops in spring 1744 to that which had prevailed at the same time a year before, Buchanan observes, "When the weather become dry & warm, the ground dry, Complaints were much the same as last Season, but having little or no fatigue, the weather was not so excessive hot, they were neither so frequent nor violent." The fact that in general the troops were inured to the march also promoted health: "The men were accustomed to a Campn life." Significantly too, they "were always supplyed with plenty of good provision." Still another factor that promoted health was habitation. According to Buchanan, during the march the men had "abundance of Straw, lived well & made huts to shed themselves from the Sun, which we never did in Germany on account of frequent marching, nor did the Country afford such plenty of wood, nor durst we make free with it as in Flanders" [p. 307]. The huts allowed for free circulation of air—a marked contrast to the sweltering tents that Buchanan condemned.

Anticipating the advice that Richard Brocklesby would enunciate in 1764, in his influential *Oeconomical and Medical Observations*, Buchanan puts forward in "Regimental Practice" a few rules for maintaining health when the army was encamped. It was, he argues, important to choose a healthful campsite, to keep it clean, and occasionally to shift ground:

> If we continue ... long in one Camp our <men> grow lousy & itchy ... their straw should be often changed; the old always burnt & not thrown as litter to the horses ... if we remaine a long time in the same Camp, there's an ugly smell, from the horse Dung, & large swarms of flies become troublesome, especially in hot weather. if the ground be wettish, with many ditches of stagnating water, fish ponds, &c: the water stinks in hot weather & is useless, being full of frogs Spawn &c: [pp. 323, 325]

Like most of his contemporaries, Buchanan looked to the non-naturals both to preserve health and to restore it. The Flemish were in his opinion typically healthier than were the English, in part because they enjoyed sufficient rest and good air: "Playes & other entertainments are never so late as in London. the Gentlemen keep themselves warmer than at home. some from prudence in preserving health, others from the custome of the Country ... here is no coale smoake" [pp. 241,

243]. Likewise he witnessed patients recovering from ague "without Bark or any other febrifuge medecine, which was entirely owing to a warmer & dryer air" [p. 35].

One of the factors that Buchanan frequently notes as he compares the health of different groups is diet. He reports, for example, that jaundice was "hardly known amongst the towns people ... they eat very little meat, living much on vegetables" [p. 135]. It appears that he favored simple diets that were vegetable oriented. In Flanders, he writes, "Consumptive people are more healthie ... live much on vegetables, all garden herbs being in great abundance & good of their kind" [p. 165]. At another point he observes, "Our Officers were more healthie abroad than at home ... this proceeds from a lighter dyet; in England solid meats are most common[;] here a light soup is always the first dish ... nor are dressed Suppers much in fashion" [p. 241].

Buchanan also considered the issue of drink—specifically, which alcoholic beverages the men drank, how much, and how regularly—in relation to disease. Indeed, alcohol consumption figures frequently in his observations, suggesting that he was interested in the possibility of linkage. He reports, for example, that the only man who died in an outbreak of pleuretic fever was an "old Drammer" [p. 109]. A soldier who died costive, Buchanan observes, "was remarkably Sprightly, but from bad example has learned to drink Drams. was often Drunk & it was thought his inside was burnt up" [p. 145]. He judges alcohol abuse to be an occasional cause of various diseases, including dropsy [p. 150] and colic [p. 235]. And in his estimation, inflammatory fever was dangerous only to heavy drinkers [p. 102].

Nevertheless, on the subject of drink, Buchanan provides a mixed message. Wine, particularly the lighter ones, he considered to be salubrious. Malt liquor, if not too strong, he generally approved of, even when it was drunk in excess. Discussing the dissection of a drunkard; he notes that the liver was not burnt or dry, and he ascribes this to the fact that the dead man generally drank malt liquor [p. 331]. He believed that the overall health of the Flemish had much to do with their choice of liquor and their overall sobriety, for they were not guilty of "any excess of drinking at taverns, it being customary to retire to each others private Lodgings & pass the evening in a Sober manner; here are no country rambles ... light French wines are drunk dayly instead of Strong Port ... here is no ... strong malt liquor" [pp. 241, 243]. However, other observations in "Regimental Practice" suggest that he was cautious in linking disease to drunkenness. As has been noted, he dismisses the claim that gin drinking provoked an outbreak of flux in 1745. "None of our drunke fellows catched <it>," he writes of the yellow fever epidemic of 1743 [p. 63]. In relation to ague, he observes, "Drinking Gin & Spirituous Liquors are said to occasion this distemper; our foot Guards are remarkable for this taste, yet not much Subject to the desease, and all our drunken fellows have escaped the distemper ... it was almost universal with the garrison at Bruges, especially where their barracks were moist & cold" [p. 33]. He even discounts the common—and, it would turn out, correct—opinion that indulgence in strong, sweet wines encouraged gout: "Gouty Officers avoid drinking French wines, for fear of giving them the Gout. but in Flanders it's the only wine they drink, particularly Burgundy, Hermitage & acknowledge they never were so healthy. & in our Dutch cantoonment French claret was drunk dayly & that freely, yet I don't remember many Gouty complaints" [p. 163]. Looking back over the service of the Blues on the Continent, Buchanan observes, "The Drunken fellows have been remarkably healthie since we came abroad" [p. 329]. He adds, however, "when taken ill, their distempers are more violent, & some dye suddenly" [p. 331].

At least in "Regimental Practice," Buchanan does not moralize in discussing venereal disease. He views the disease itself as discouraging promiscuity, noting, "When the men have been often in for it, they are more cautious in their intrigues" [p. 197].

Buchanan was more consistent in his attitude toward exercise. He comments in his journal that sedentary soldiers were most prone to illness while the army was in winter quarters; and that he did not believe that garrison duty provided meaningful exercise [p. 333]. Officers, he observes, were prone to indulgence when in winter quarters [p. 335]. Buchanan notes the negative impact on health of a sedentary life. He warmly advocates horseback riding as exercise, sometimes pointing up detrimental health consequences for those who neglected it [pp. 149, 169, 241, 335]. In general, he endorses exercise as an antidote to over-indulgence [pp. 133, 135]. Reflective of his overall tendency toward moderate therapies is his advocacy of lifestyle adjustments in treating consumption, while many contemporaries were more reliant on drugs [p. 167].

Treating Disease

Beyond questioning the patients regarding their symptoms, Buchanan diagnosed diseases and traced their progress through checking signs and symptoms that were readily observable. He was, however, selective in what he looked for: "I seldom examine the Troopers urine, they having no proper conveniency to keep it, and think I can form a better judgement from their voice, looks & breathing, than from their pulse or Urine" [p. 99].

Eighteenth-century British therapeutics grew from the firm foundation of Thomas Sydenham. He, far more than any other individual, shaped the methods by which disease was understood and treated. In the corpus of his published writings —small by comparison to those of a number of far less important figures—there were many diseases that he did not discuss, but even in these cases the broad rules that he laid down often had influence. It is unclear whether Buchanan read any of his works. In "Regimental Practice" he does mention that he treats smallpox "after Sydenham's manner" [p. 45], and he endorses Sydenham's recommendation of horseback riding as therapy for consumption [p. 167]. But the views expressed by Sydenham were in both cases so well known that Buchanan could have picked them up by word of mouth.

For some illnesses, Buchanan recognized no treatment as effective. With respect to the common cold, he observes in his journal, "This is one of the most common Deseases & most difficult to cure in many cases. & people are surprized we cannot cure a cold for which every body has his own favorite medecine, but dissection often Shows them to be incurable" [p. 127]. And while some contemporaries were sanguine about curing dropsy, he reports, "the common method of cure attempted, but never succeeded, & I never saw a real Dropsy cured tho it may be palliated by medecines, tapping &c." [p. 149]. In the main, however, Buchanan was an optimist, confident that most diseases could be cured and that he could play a major role in this.

Buchanan appears to have favored drugs that were moderate in action. When a rapid purge was not essential, he preferred diet to drugs as a laxative, noting in his journal that in treating smallpox patients, "I endeavour to procure a stool every other day, by dyet or Clister, & by so doing many bad Symptoms are prevented, but would rather have it by Dyet so as to empty the whole tube of the Guts, & for this purpose I advise roasted apples, stewed pears, currant or Plumb: Gruelle, now & then a draught of whey, &c:" [pp. 45, 47].

In the course of "Regimental Practice," Buchanan cites 111 drugs or unnamed medicinal preparations that he definitely or probably used—in a number of cases, he notes that others used them, as well—plus 66 that were used by others, but not by him, at least not in the instances that he mentions. In addition to particular remedies, he occasionally refers to drugs only by category: "digestives," "mercurials," "saponaceous medicines," and the like. The number of remedies that he made use of is surprisingly large. In his period, practitioners, often after an initial phase of trial and error, tended to focus on a short list of drugs that they applied rather broadly.[54] Even though, as of the start of his chronicle in September 1742, Buchanan had already been a regimental surgeon for more than eight years, he was clearly experimenting and was furthermore adjusting his choices in accordance with a set of variables, such as the nature and intensity of symptoms and the condition, perhaps also the preferences, of the patient.

Most of the remedies that Buchanan specifies shared the names of official drugs, as they were set forward in the *Pharmacopeia Londinensis* and the *Pharmacopeia Edinburgensis*. This may not mean, however, that they were always prepared according to the recipes of London or Edinburgh, for the army had its own formulas. There were, first of all, the drugs that Buchanan refers to as "nostrums." Buchanan mentions using fourteen of these. While not always stating an opinion regarding their effectiveness, he writes favorably of those that he does assess. The army's mercurial pill he characterizes as "the best I know," and he states that the

[54] For example, while as a naval surgeon Thomas Robertson had more than 60 drugs in his medical chest, he apparently made use of only a few, employing these repeatedly: William N. Boog Watson, "Thomas Robertson, Naval Surgeon, 1793–1828." BHM, 46 (1972), p. 136.

liniment for venereal ulcers was capable of "dissolving them insensibly without pain & [I] have been often surprized at its good success" [pp. 177, 185].

Beyond the remedies that Buchanan mentions, there were many others that were prepared in accordance with a standard army formula. A manuscript "Dispensatory for the Army Hospitals," which was fixed as standard by Cumberland's order, provides recipes for 45 drugs, most of them directed by their names to the treatment of particular diseases and symptoms—*Enema Dysentericum* and *Infusum Pectorale*, for example.[55] It appears to have been prepared in March 1746, although it is possible that this did not take place until the following winter.[56]

The dispensatory suggests that the drugs were prepared according to the recipes of either London or the army, but not Edinburgh. It includes no references to Edinburgh, but a number to London. It is also noteworthy that George Garnier, the apothecary-general and one of the co-signers of a statement approving the formulas in the dispensatory, was a member of the Society of Apothecaries of London.[57] He was responsible for providing regimental surgeons with their medical chests and for preparing the compound drugs that were included. It is probable that drugs that had the same names as those that were included in the pharmacopoeias of London or Edinburgh were routinely prepared from London recipes. However, when apothecaries in army hospitals prepared compound drugs on the request of the regimental surgeons, the surgeons appear to have had some leeway in ordering. Buchanan appears to have had a preference for the Edinburgh recipe for *decoctum nitrosum*, for he specifies this version in two prescriptions noted in "Regimental Practice" [pp. 62, 83].

The core coverage of Buchanan's manuscript, 1742–45, just misses the landmark fifth edition of the London pharmacopoeia in 1746. It must therefore be assumed that, except in the cases noted above, the compound drugs referred to by Buchanan were prepared in accordance with the recipes set out in the most recent edition of the pharmacopoeia, which had been published in 1721. Although there had been some paring in this edition, the intensity of revision did not even

---

[55] Royal Archives, Windsor Castle, Cumberland Papers, Box 2.26, pp. 4–10. Apparently on Cumberland's authority, in 1747 John Theobald published the recipes in translation and discussed their uses: Medulla Medicinae Universae: or, A New Compendious Dispensatory. Compiled at the Command of His Royal Highness the Duke, For the Use of the Military Hospital Abroad, during the late War. By the King's Physicians and Surgeons, the Surgeon-General, and Apothecary-General, to the Army.

[56] The manuscript is in fact dated "9 March 1745," but the reference is probably to 1745/46.

[57] George Garnier (1703–63) gained the freedom of the society on 7 July 1735, after completing an apprenticeship to his father, Isaac: Guildhall Library, London, Manuscript Section, Records of the Society of Apothecaries, Freedom Books, #8206/2, p. 33. On Isaac Garnier's death, he succeeded him as apothecary-general, gaining his commission 7 March 1736: Johnston's Roll, I, 1 (#8), 9 (#161). Note also Arthur E. Garnier, The Chronicles of the Garniers of Hampshire during Four Centuries, 1530–1900 (London: Jarrold, 1900), pp. 14, 21.

approach that of 1746, when hundreds of recipes were virtually rewritten and many compound drugs were unceremoniously deleted.

Nevertheless, the evidence in his journal suggests that Buchanan's practice was oriented toward newer medicines. He makes rather little use of drugs, simple or compound, that appear to have been declining in popularity. He does use theriac, one of the last galenicals, which was already under attack and would be eliminated from the London pharmacopoeia in 1788. However, he appears to have employed it as a mild opiate and sudorific, rather than because he was impressed by the traditional claim that it was effective against pestilence [pp. 21, 85, 113]. He was an enthusiastic supporter of the army's experiment with cerated glass of antimony, a drug that was hailed by some as a specific for dysentery, for as he observes with apparent satisfaction, "our Allies knew nothing of this medecine, so treated it with small Doses Ipecacaon: & Rhabarb. & some of our Surgeons do the same, never making tryale of Vitr. Cerat: Antimon: & probably the good success from it may be in a great measure owing to my persisting in its use" [p. 282]. In assessing the worth of drugs that were new or at least new to him, Buchanan notes experiments by other medical officers. These, like his own observations, might well challenge the value of traditional remedies. He reports for example that another regimental surgeon had given his men walnut pith to cure their dysentery. The pith had long been considered a specific for the disease, but the surgeon did not find it to have a positive effect [p. 291].

Like Sydenham, whose advocacy of opiates was so warm that he was known as *Opiophilus*, Buchanan strongly endorsed opium. He nevertheless recognized that there was significant controversy over when, even whether, to use it, going so far as to write, "in England there's a universal prejudice against Opiates, in camp practice I have used them more freely than any other medicine" [p. 59]. Recalling how he had treated the mild fevers that had struck many soldiers in the spring of 1743, Buchanan reports, "a day's rest was the best medecine, & the opiate the best cordiale, procuring a good night's rest, enabled them for the nixt day's fatigue. I used Opium freely & from seeing it's good effects, became a favorite medecine" [p. 60]. Similarly, of the effects of pure opium in the treatment of rheumatism, he writes, "Opiates were of the greatest service, especially when given in large Doses ... a good night's rest was always procured & sweats promoted, & seldom or never observed any bad effects from this free use of Opium, but am convinced it's the most universal medecine for soldiers. it became a universal practice, & the pure Opium is equal to any of it's preparations" [p. 301].

No less than the opiates, Buchanan exalted bark. In the case of ague, he asserts, "it's needless to enquire for a more certaine remedy than the Simple Barke, if the disease once form into a regular Ague, I am certaine it will cure and never saw it faile" [p. 29]. He defends bark against the criticism that it caused jaundice [pp. 135, 137].[58] By the 1740s however, the value of bark in medicine was well established, so his advocacy of it would not have been unusual.

Buchanan recognized that drugs were often falsely credited with cures that were merely coincidental to their use. He observes in his journal, "if worms are voided during the course of any medecine, it's always looked upon as a good Vermefuge" [p. 233]. Patterns of success impressed him, however. It appears that, like many contemporaries, he came to support inoculation as a means of reducing mortality associated with smallpox. In reference to an epidemic in Stafford in 1756, he notes that none of the twenty-seven patients who had been inoculated died [interleaf pp. 61-62 in "RP" Ms.].

The marketing of a nostrum could bring a practitioner significant income and notoriety, though sometimes at the cost of envy and vituperation from his peers. Like many medical men, Buchanan hit on formulas that he regarded as effective, but he chose not to conceal them. He reports that he had successfully treated inflamed eyes with a solution of milk, water, and brandy and added, "had I concealed it as a nostrum, it might have passed for a famous Eye water" [p. 248].

"Regimental Practice" deals with horses as well as their riders. As surgeon to a cavalry regiment, Buchanan was expected to assist the farriers in treating sick and injured horses. It was not until the 1790s that veterinarians were added to the establishment of horse regiments. In any case, veterinary medicine received little attention in eighteenth-century Britain, though a number of works were written on farrying.[59]

Just as Buchanan was quick to discount legends regarding human health issues when his observations did not accord with them, so was he prone to challenging acquired wisdom about horses. In Flanders he observed, "I have heared some Gentlemen curious in horses say that a necessary house near the Stable was dangerous for horses, that the smell of it would breake their wind. but here it's customary to have them in the corner of the Stable, & it's rare to see a broken winded horse" [p. 245].

It appears that Buchanan was often called upon to advise farriers who were attached to the Blues. As he saw it, they were typically unable to handle problems that were not familiar from the civilian world: "our Farriers were strangers to

---

[58] On the other hand, he does report the case of a woman who developed jaundice after treating herself with bark [p. 75].

[59] Although as Elector George III encouraged the founding of a veterinary college in Hanover, he did not do so in Britain. Nevertheless, there were some significant developments in veterinary medicine during the latter half of the century, culminating in the founding of the London Veterinary College in 1791. As Louise Hill Curth has noted, horses had traditionally received special treatment, and members of the Company of Farriers were the elite among animal doctors, followed by others who treated horses: "The Care of the Brute Beast: Animals and the Seventeenth-century Medical Market-place," Social History of Medicine, 15 (2002), pp. 375, 382–6; note also Ernest A. Gray, "John Hunter and Veterinary Medicine," Medical History, 1 (1957), pp. 38–9.

Gunshot wounds & I treated some wounded horses much in the same manner as I did the men" [p. 277]. That Buchanan treated the wounds of horses as he would have those of their riders reflected his general perspective. With the exception of "crib-biting," he saw equine diseases to have their human equivalents [p. 316], and this suggested analogous therapy. But just as his therapeutics in the treatment of human diseases was characteristically moderate, so were the methods that he tended to employ in treating horses, and in this respect he appears to have been far from most of the farriers, for they used old remedies that were often harsh.[60] Buchanan reports, "Cracked heels are dressed by the Farriers with an Oynt of Verdigrease, & appear to be too sharp, rather fretting than healing. I use Basilicon with a small portion of Ungt. Aegyptiac., & is then digestive, cleaning & healing" [p. 253]. Similarly, while noting that it had become a common practice to purge horses that were exhausted from campaigning, he observes, "My horses had no medecines nor were they blooded, stood in a cool Stable, had dayly exercise & recovered well" [p. 253].

Buchanan had evident sympathy for the horses of the army. According to him, in the wake of Fontenoy, "The wounded horses would not foresake their Regmts though they had lost their Riders, & followed so long as they could walk, & some had only three legs to stand on" [p. 277]. He appears to have viewed the fashion of docking as not only unnecessary but injurious.

> English horses for want of their tails are greatly tormented with flies during the warm weather; fatigue themselves with kicking & stamping, wear out their Shoes, breake & Spoyle the ground; tossing their heads backwards to beat off the flies, lose their forrage. the fatigue is so much that it makes them sweat as they stand at the picket, & fall off their flesh. None of our Allies docke their horses & are allowed a smaller ratiate than ours, by two or three pounds of hay, yet are fatter & look better than ours by the latter end of the Campn. [p. 317]

His sensitivity regarding the horses reflects a common theme implicit in "Regimental Practice": Buchanan appears to have been a compassionate individual, and this drove the method that he used to treat disease. The therapy that characterized his practice was typically moderate, standing in sharp contrast to more aggressive, heroic methods.[61]

Theory in Practice

As has been noted, Buchanan regularly tested theories and discounted many on the basis of his observations. But these theories were small scale, usually relating

---

[60] The farriers' influence in medical matters was not limited to the horses. According to Buchanan, they sold eyewaters to the troops; "RP" Ms., p. 247.

[61] For context, see Kopperman, "The Drive toward More Moderate Therapies," pp. 266–9.

to the cause, nature, or cure of a particular disease: whether fresh fruit caused dysentery, whether ague could be cured by terror, and the like. They played out within a broad conceptual framework that informed both his understanding of disease and his method of treating it.

In a period when "empiric" was always used pejoratively among regular medical men—for it described a quack or fringe practitioner, who proceeded without method—"empirical" was often allowed a positive connotation. Medical professionals were supposed to challenge traditional beliefs, particularly on the basis of observation and experiment. On the other hand, if they challenged a paradigm that spoke to the nature, causes, and treatment of disease, they could expect criticism, and if they tore down a popular system without offering an alternative, vituperation was certain. Like many of his contemporaries, Buchanan was to a degree oriented toward empiricism, but he was by no means an empiric.

Insofar as it related to the broad strategy of treating disease, Buchanan's medical theory can be explained in terms of two complementary paradigms, both of which dated back to the Greeks and were commonplace, though not standard, in eighteenth-century British medicine. One was that nature controlled the entire process of sickness and health, and that when confronted with a disease condition it was the duty of the physician to interpret and support the tendencies of nature as it attempted to provide a cure. The second was that there were essentially two types of disease, which for simplicity we may denominate "high" and "low," and that the therapy that was called for in the treatment of a disease in the former category differed markedly, even diametrically, from what was appropriate to the latter. Symptoms that characterized high diseases included a strong, rapid pulse, fever, and inflammation. Low diseases were marked by weak pulse and prostration. In general, the high diseases were seen to be the product of an overcharged, overstimulated system, while low diseases were accounted to debility and insufficient stimulation. Although the boundaries might seem to be clear, many diseases, such as smallpox, passed through a series of stages and appeared at times high, at times low, which meant that the treatment that was commonly thought wise in one stage might be considered dangerous in another.

Like so many contemporaries, when treating a patient Buchanan attempted to detect and respond to the signs provided by nature. With reference to men who suffered from pleuretic fevers in 1743, Buchanan notes that "Some naturally inclined to sweat which was promoted" [p. 113]. But unless the signs were clear, the practitioner was to proceed with caution: "Fevers often attempt to throw themselves off thro the Pores of the skin, breaking out in sweats, & if naturale, are of great service & often compleat the cure. when I perceive a naturale inclination to sweat I encourage it by drinking freely of the above drinks, encreasing the quantity of wine & covering warm, which ought to be done with prudence for fear of encreasing the fever" [p. 83]. By the same token, he writes, nature was not to be coerced: "One should be cautious of forcing sweats at this time" [p. 85]. Supporting the system was all important: "in all Sicknesses it should be the principale care of a physician to preserve the Stomach in good order. for when that failes, adieu to all remedies, & it is often spoiled by drugs rather than the distemper" [p. 105].

Another insight into Buchanan's thought process lies in the queries that he puts forward in two instances. When a fever victim was autopsied, his lungs were found to be filled with blood and marked by black spots. Buchanan ponders the results in his journal: "N:B: this patient had always a tickling dry cough, & pectoral medecines never had any good effect. did it proceed from the largenes of the heart interrupting the motion of the Lungs? as all men have different complexions, features, make &c: nature seems to have observed the same rule with regard to the inside, for we observe great variety as to it's size form &c: hence probably different tempers, passions, &c." [p. 69]. Later, a trooper, who was in hospital being treated for a fever, appeared to be recovering, but suddenly he began to experience sudden and violent pain in his left leg and he died in agony the following morning. The leg then swelled and turned livid, and on dissection it was found to contain gelatinous matter. Buchanan wonders, "Quaer: 1mo. was this an attempt of nature to form a criticale absess here. 2do. would scarifications with warm digestives been of any use." [p. 331]. Clearly, Buchanan was seeking to interpret the signs of nature and to treat disease accordingly.

It was widely assumed that if patients craved a particular food or beverage, nature was speaking through them. Buchanan took this into consideration in determining diet: "Negus is a favourite drink with our men of which they drink freely ... having a pleasant smell, it's extreamely agreable to the Sick; holding tamarinds in the mouth or sucking oranges greatly quenches thirst; the mouth should be often washed with common drink in order to relax the Glands; all drinks to be drunk moderately warm & freely. nature demands it" [p. 83].

In formulating therapy, Buchanan displayed a respect for nature. He likewise observed the boundary between high and low diseases. His practice on bloodletting illustrates this well. The use of bloodletting in therapy and the quantity of blood taken appears to have been on the rise during the first half of the eighteenth century. Although venesection had been incorporated into European medicine for centuries, many major authorities had allowed for it only in a limited range of circumstances, and even then in small quantities. Sydenham had, however, boosted bloodletting, allowing it a key place in the treatment of many diseases and prescribing it as the central therapy for some. In Buchanan's time, several of the most influential physicians, Pringle and John Huxham among them, went still further, advocating bleeding, often in large quantities, even in circumstances where it had traditionally not been used.[62]

[62] John Ball wrote, "Though most authors, as well ancient as modern, generally agree, that Malignant Fevers by no means admit of bleeding, yet the ingenious and successful practitioners, Sydenham and Astruc, indiscriminately order it in all cases; and Huxham and Pringle allow it may be performed, with advantage, under certain circumstances, especially in the beginning": The Modern Practice of Physic: or a Method of judiciously Treating the Several Disorders incident to the Human Body (London: A. Millar, 1760), I, 120.

Buchanan held with contemporary practice when he asserted that it was necessary to bleed victims of rheumatism, because their pulse was "quick & full" [p. 299]. Particular diseases prompted him to bleed his patients aggressively. If he suspected quinsy, "on the first complaint I bleed largely, even though the pulse be not feverish" [p. 121]. Furthermore, in at least one instance, he bled in a situation that did not, in the opinion of some contemporaries, call for it: "I have blooded many Troopers in the first access [of ague], & don't think it retarded the cure" [p. 41].

Generally, however, Buchanan was cautious in letting blood. When fatigued men wished to be bled, he advised against it [p. 327]. During an outbreak of slow fever in 1743 he found "pulse so low that bleeding did not seem proper" [p. 293]. By holding back in this instance, he followed common practice. Perhaps more than many contemporaries, he was sensitive to the danger of excessive bleeding: "When the pulse sinks from bleeding too freely it's not easely raised by medicines." [p. 119].

"Regimental Practice" suggests that Buchanan did not let blood as a matter of course. Venesection had to have a purpose. With reference to the men who suffered from gripes and purging in 1742, he observes, "seldom attended with fever, of course no occasion for bleedings" [p. 19]. He appears to have been reluctant to bleed in treating diseases that contemporaries would have considered "malignant" or "putrid," notably remittent or continued fevers, such as typhus. On occasion, his practice was probably influenced by common opinion among medical officers. In the treatment of yellow fever, he reports, "bleeding was thought hurtfull" [p. 63]. But apparently he bled less than did many of his colleagues, a case in point being reflected in his account of an outbreak of "fever with eruptions" in early 1743: "with some Physicians bleeding was much in vogue, in a few days the Patient lost 60, 70, 80, 90, Ounces, which was attended with bad success for few recovered. I seldom blooded unless difficult breathing or Stich &c: forced me, & all my men did well" [pp. 117, 119].

While Buchanan bled cautiously, he routinely used expellant drugs. More often than not, he initiated treatment with an emetic. Vomiting was also a standard in prophylactic medicine. Practitioners who believed that they were falling ill routinely attempted to forestall the disease by taking a vomit [e.g., p. 293]. Buchanan did not prescribe emetics as a matter of course. He mentions, for example, that when treating gripes he did not administer them unless the patient was squeamish [p. 21]. Nevertheless, he saw them as useful in cases where not all contemporaries did. While observing that "Some object" to the use of expellant drugs on fever patients who had not eaten for several days and whose vomit and stool were clear, he defends his practice: "we see dayly good effects from a vomite, tho the water come up as clear as when drunk; great advantages may be obtained from purgative medicines tho the Stools are not excrementitious, there being a large discharge from the Glands of the Gutts. so in a cold the head is greatly relieved by a large discharge of clear thin water thro the nostrills, though no snot passes." [pp. 79, 81].

The practice portrayed in Buchanan's manuscript possesses a coherence that had grown from his earlier education, his readings, and eight prior years of service as a regimental surgeon. It is not, however, dogmatic, nor is it stagnant. Buchanan experimented with new techniques and new remedies for treating the diseases that he encountered while serving the Blues in Flanders. He was interested in the potential for new inventions to improve medicine. Of a case reported in "Regimental Practice," he observes that the patient's collar bone was "easely broke & as easely reduced, yet there's no credite got by it, for its not easely keeped in its place & the Surgn is blamed for not setting it well, the bandage seldom presses on the part, but too much under the Armpits & becomes uneasy to the patient. I wish a proper Screw could be contrived for this purpose" [p. 223]. And it appears that his interest in medical discoveries continued after he returned to civilian practice. In 1766, the board of the Staffordshire General Infirmary noted that staff had requested the purchase of electrical equipment, and it approved the order.[63] Very likely it was Buchanan who, as the chief medical officer of the infirmary, put forward this request. The type of equipment ordered was just coming into fashion, being used to treat palsy and other problems that were thought to respond well to stimulation. By advocating for it, Buchanan was keeping his practice up to date.

---

[63] Staffs RO, D685/2/1, (#36).

Notes on Transcription

Superscript to mark elisions, as in "Sept^{r}," will generally be brought down to the line; when Buchanan abbreviates book sizes with superscript, as in "8°," I will as well, to avoid confusion.

Angle brackets (<>) are used to indicate that a word or phrase is inserted interlinearly in the manuscript; if Buchanan marks the place of insertion, this will be indicated with a caret (^).

Buchanan does not always mark off ellipses in quotations, and when he does so he usually uses a double line (=); in either case, I will indicate breaks in quoted material with ellipses (… or ….).

All translations from Latin appear in braces ({}). I will embolden and italicize the translations and for the most part set them off from the text. The formulas that Buchanan provides, as well as some short quoted phrases, will be embedded in the text, as Buchanan has them. Buchanan generally incorporates prose quotations into his text and does not set them off except (occasionally) by quotation marks or (more often) by a diagonal or vertical stroke. Poetry he often sets off, but generally if he quotes a single line he does so within the text.

The letter thorn (þ; in eighteenth-century hand, often indistinguishable from a y) is transcribed as "th."

Following convention, Buchanan routinely concludes each verso page with the first word of the next verso, setting it off in the lower right-hand corner; I omit this.

In the footnotes and throughout the introduction, it is my practice to date the year from 1 January (e.g., 15 March 1743, rather than 1742–43).

Buchanan sometimes uses dashes to close paragraphs, or to extend a line of text to the margin. I omit these when they are superfluous and otherwise replace them with periods.

Entries on the verso page usually appear opposite the points they are cited or that they qualify; in the transcription, bracketed notations will indicate their place on the page, unless Buchanan makes this clear by a reference mark (invariably a letter) in superscript.

Regimental Practice.

or

A Short History of Diseases common to His Majesties own Royale Regiment of Horse Guards when abroad (Commonly called the Blews)

by

John Buchanan M:D: Surgeon to the Regiment.

1746.

{"[There is] no book so bad but some profit be gleaned from it"}
Plin. Epist:1. lib:3[1]

[1] Pliny, Letters 3.5. To read this, medinical recipes, and other translations in the original Latin, the reader may consult *Theory and Practice*, the online version of this book.

1.

A Short History of Diseases common to His Majesties own Royale Regiment of Horse Guards, commonly called the Blews, when Abroad.

[*margin:* Embark at Gravesend] Par: 1st. The Regiment embarked at Gravesend Septr 1st 1742. O:S: in good health, without any remarkable accident to man or horse; had a good passage to Ostend, being only three days at sea with fair weather:

[*margin:* Officers & men are seasick] the most part of Officers and men were sea:sick, purging and vomiting freely. The soldiers were allowed by the publick, one pound bread, half a pound salt butter, and one quarter pound cheese for dayly dyet, with two quarts small beer, or half a pint brandy, for drink; which was not a sufficient quantity, the weather being extreamely

2. [*facing p. 1; blank*]

3. [*continuing from p. 1*]

hot we found it necessary to give three quarts <beer> for which extraordinary quart the commanding Officer gave his receipt to the Master of the Ship.[2] Officers servants had the same allowance: Officers laid in their own fresh provisions and had as much ship beer as they pleased. The ship air was very warm and suffocating from heat of the weather and breath of the horses, and drought was a general complaint. such as were not sea-sick were costive from their dyet & air.

[*margin:* Horses not affected by the motion of the ship.] Our horses were not in the least affected from the motion of the ship: fed as usual, but were not more greedy of water; and such as were broken winded were much worse when some time aboard:

[*margin:* Method of keeping at sea] we opened the ship-ports to cool and air them. we wet our hay and corn well,

4. see Military orders & instructions for preserving the health of soldiers when on board Transports contained in a Pamphelet entitled, a Journal of the Campaign on the coast of France. 1758. p.13. &c.[3]

5. [*continuing from p. 3*]

which <was> refreshing and cooling to the horses; watered and fed three times a day, viz: at six, at Noon, and at night; which was three quarters a

[2] The officer referred to by Buchanan was probably Lieut.-Col. Gregory Beake (cf. below, n. 10).

[3] *Journal of the Campaign on the Coast of France, 1758* (London: J. Townsend, 1758), esp. pp. 13–15.

day; as the Government's allowance is a peck, we saved the other quarter for the use of our troops when a share.

[*margin:* method of treating sick horses.] When a horse sickens by heat, a little water cools and relieves him;

[*margin:* Bleeding of great use.] if unease at the head, tossing it backwards and forwards, biting and catching at the Manger or collar reins, then it's absolutely necessary to bleed him immediately, or the consequence will be very bad; and some horses were lost for want of this help; if he cannot be conveniently blooded at the neck, let him be blooded in the mouth, when he has lost a sufficient quantity, rub the part with flower in order to stop it. – horse's ears

6. [*facing p. 5; blank*]

7. [*continuing from p. 5*]
to be often pulled, and heads rubed, which refreshes them greatly and takes off their shyness. a quart blood should be taken away the first halting day[4] after the landing. as they stood some dayes on their own Dung and Stale. their hoofs were softer & moister, and easely lost their shoes.

[*margin:* Disembark at Ostend.] Par: 2d. Disembark at Ostend, Septr 4th, free of accidents.

[*margin:* slight complaints at Disembarking] some troopers not being used to walk across the ship ropes broke their <u>shins</u>, which they <cured> by washing with brandy; only <two> were so bad as to be under my care; was obliged to poultice, digest, incarn &c: such as had been sick at sea were now faint and weake; others overheated themselves in disembarking the horses; all were obliged to lye on straw in an open warehouse, by their

8. [*facing p. 7; blank*]

9. [*continuing from p. 7*]:

horses, having only ship allowance (Par: 1st.) for provision, were obliged to eat such things as were easily got, viz: [*crossed:* such as fruits] Pears, Plumbs, Grapes &c: of which they were very fond, and eat heartely.

> {**"Only a stomach that seldom feels hunger scorns things common."**}
>
> Hor: Sat:2. lb 2. v.37.[5]

and proved the beginning of many complaints,

---

4 A day on which the army remained in camp and did not march.

5 Horace, Satires 2.2.38 [not 37].

{"For when the veins are empty one should admit nothing to them that is not mild."}

Hor: Sat:6. lib:2 v.25.[6] –

[*margin:* March to Bruges] Par: 3. Many complained next morning of catching cold, were griped; for which they drank a pennyworth of Gin or Brandywyne, and marched to Bruges that day being cold & wet;

[*margin:* great difference twixt the English & Flemish quarters.] were billited in publick <& private> houses, neitheir dyet nor fire provided as in England, nor forage for their horses, which they were obliged to bring on their backs from the Bylanders in the wet; were at great loss for want of the language, & obliged

10. [*facing p. 9; blank*]

11. [*continuing from p. 9*]:
to eat as (Par:2). now began to drink punch to keep themselves warm –

{"Diseases do not suddenly seize men, but gather gradually before bursting forth."}

Hip: de vict: rat: lb: 1. Sect: 6.[7]

[*margin:* March to Ghent.] Par: 4. Next day had a long march to Ghent;

[*margin:* the legs swell on long marching] many of the men had swelled legs from being so long on horseback, especially such as were fat & corpulent, which obliged them to stay in their barracks some dayes, & soon complain'd of grieps & looseness: as this increased their legs decreased; nor did I endeavour to stop it until they became faint an [*sic*] weake, and Pulv: Rhabarb: scr. ii. with Pil: Math: h: s: repeated twice or thrice with Decoct: alb: cum Gum: Arabic: compleated the cure, and living on mutton broth thickened with Rye[a] Such as had hurt their shins as in Par: 2. were now worse than at first from the

12.

[a] **{"In disorders of the bowels, and in vomits that are spontaneous, if what is purged is of such a sort as should be purged, one profits and endures easily. But if not, the contrary comes to pass. Likewise with artificial evacuations, if what takes place ought to take place, he may profit and easily bear it. If not, the contrary. Therefore, consider location, season, age and disease, to see if this treatment ought to be used or not."}** Hip: Aphorism: No. 2. lib: ii. s:ii.[8]

---

[6] Hor. Sat. 2.4 [not 6].25–6.

[7] Hippocrates, Regimen, 1.2.62–4.

[8] Hippocrates, Aphorism 1.2 [not 2.2].

13. [*continuing from p. 11*]:
pressure of the boot, & long march; were easily cured by poultices of white bread and milk or turnep &c.[b]

[*margin:* In Baracks at Ghent] Par: 5. All are now in Barracks, ordered to Boyle their kettle and mess regularly; all provisions being as good and as cheap as at home, they may live well; their only complaint is want of fire, having no more allowed by the town than what is necessary to boyle the kettle[a]; and that is not near sufficient to air the barracks, which have been empty houses sometime, of consequence are damp, especially such as are near the canals; all have been lately white washed & are scarcely dry. two men lye in one bed on Matrasses of coarse flax, are well enough covered, but have no curtains.

[*margin:* Diseases in Garrison(:) The Itch] Par: 6. The first distemper that was remarkable amongst the men was the Itch, to which we were strangers when at home, (the dirty fellows exempted) but was now

14. vid. Fred: Hoffmanni Op: Med: Tom: 3. p.363. de praestantia Remediorum Domesticorum.[9]
{**"Let [soldiers] not suffer a lack of wood and may the supply of clothing not be insufficient for them; a soldier who is suffering from the cold is neither fit in health nor suitable for a campaign."**}
Vegetius de re militari lb.3 c.2.

15. [*continuing from p. 13*]
common.

[*margin:* Diseases in Garrison(:) Causes.] The men being hurried in embarking their horses and taking care of them when aboard, seasick &c: neglected to shift and keep themselves clean; our transports had carried over the foot & Dragoons might be affected, & Dyet in (Par: 1.) might produce this distemper, in curing of which the Mercuriale Ointment was the chief application, rubbing twixt the fingers, wrists & Hams; such as were obstinate were blooded & purged, taking as much Flowers of Brimstone as would lie on a Skelline, in warm milk or common treacle every morning. it declined daily, having brought it with us, few or none breeding it here.

[*margin:* None of the Officers have it, & only two of their servants.] None of the Officers had it, and only two of their servants, as

[9] Friedrich Hoffmann [Friderici Hoffmanni], *Opera omnia physico-medica denuò revisa, correcta & aucta, in sex tomos distributa* (Geneva: fratres de Tournes, 1740), V [not III; this ed. 6 vols. in 3], pt. iii, cap. 16, pp. 363–72. The chapter title translates to "Of the superiority of remedies of the household."

they dayly attended their Masters, were obliged to keep themselves clean, the Disease might be prevented.

[*margin:* not easily cured.] This disease is never to be rooted out, one man affects a whole barrack in winter Garrison and his tent Mates in the summer. Some are

16. [*facing p. 15; blank*]

17. [*continuing from p. 15*]:
cured sooner than others, and he who is last acuring gives it fresh to his Comrades.

[*margin:* Diseases in Garrison.] some are obstinate, requiring small Doses calomel, and afterwards purging it off. the Recruits often bring it with them, or breed it soon after coming.

[*margin:* the men use their own mercurial washes, which are dangerous.] some men cure themselves with Mercuriale water, Viz: boyling two pennyworth Corrosive mercury in a quart spring water into a pint, and washing the parts affected. This is too corrosive and often excoriates the parts, & sometimes raises blisters, striking the itch suddenly inwards, whence proceed violent coughs and diseases of the breast. Brampton of Collonel Beake's Troop[10] dyed consumptive from this method, as the inside of his thighs were much affected by this distemper; so the scrotum & testicles were violently swelled from this application & blistered. Unguentum nostrum ad scabiem is not so dabbing as the Mercurial Oyntment of the

18. [*facing p. 17; blank*]

19. [*continuing from p. 17*]:
shops, and is thus made, {**"Extinguish 1 oz. quicksilver with 50 drops of aqua fortis [nitric acid]; add 1 lb. lard <and 2 oz. white beeswax>; mix according to art."**} [;] this was used freely the men walking abroad dayly, keeping no regular Regimen, yet never had a bad accident, or salivation. this is more proper for the field, as not melting so soon from the heat of the weather.

---

[10] As is usually the case, only the officer commanding the unit can be identified. Lieut.-Col. Gregory Beake was commissioned a cornet in the Blues, 24 Nov. 1702. He became a major (third in command) 29 Jan. 1734 and lieut.-col. Dec. 1739. Wounded at Fontenoy, he sold his commission June 1745. He subsequently served as lieutenant-governor of Jersey and died while in this office, 19 June 1749. In his death notice in *Gentleman's Magazine*, he is described as "a brave old officer." RADCP, Box 3/47; *The Army List of 1740* (Sheffield: Sir W. C. Ling & Co., Ltd [for the Society for Army Historical Research], 1931), p. 6; *City and Court Register 1746*, p. 133; *GM*, XIX (1749), p. 284.

[*margin:* some constitutions not easely affected by the Itch] I blooded many Itchy Troopers, yet never catched the distemper. & I know a Scotch: Gentlemen who was never affected with it, though he has had many an itchy bedfellow. <vid. Hoffmanni Op: Med: Tom.2. p.426. de pustulosis et pruriginosis varii generis affectibus Cutis.>[11]

[*margin:* Grieps and Purging.] Par: 7. The complaints from Grieps & purging were very common soon after we came into Garrison, tho frequent not dangerous, were some days ill before they applyed to me, treating themselves with burnt Gin.

[*margin:* Method of cure] the method in Par: 4 always succeeded; there was never any blood, the stools whitish, slimie, & frothy,seldom attended with fever, of course no occasion for bleedings[;] the stomach was

20. [*facing p. 19; blank*]

21. [*continuing from p. 19*]:
seldom disordered therefor seldom used vomits, but if any squeameshnes the Ipecacoan was ordered.

[*margin:* Grieps often continue after the flux] Grieps often remained after the flux, a Dose Ther: Andromach h:s: drinking something warm was the best medecine, or Opiates in large doses[x] in England there's a universal prejudice against Opiates, in camp practice I have used them more freely than any other medicine, & never observed any bad consequence attending them[a]. Nixt spring complaints of this nature were frequent & treated in the same manner with the same success.

[*margin:* Causes. from drinking white Beer] Upon asking what occasioned this Distemper I was told by some, they believed it proceeded from drinking White Beer, I advised them to abstain from Beer & drink small milk punch.

{"For that region's wines I put out of court."}
Hor: Ep. 15. lb. i. v:16.

upon tryale all agreed it was a wholesome liquor. white Beer might promote the Desease by not being

22.

[x]vid: Huxham de Aere et morbis Epidemius. Lond. Vol.1. 1752. Prolegom: p.24. **{"In my Opinion, there should be now and then also interposed some gentle Laxative to carry off the bilious Corruption: This indeed**

---

11 "Of pustulous and pruriginous affections of the skin, of various kinds": Hoffmann, *Opera omnia physico-medica*, III, 426; cf. Friedrich Hoffman, *A System of the Practice of Medicine: From the Latin of Dr. Hoffman*, trans. William Lewis, rev. Andrew Duncan (London: J. Murray, 1783), II, 460.

provident Nature often effects by a Diarrhoea, Cholera, or Dysentery, which a seasonable Dose of Rhubarb, now and then administered, might have altogether prevented, and yet relieved Nature as well."}[12]

[a]Young on Opium. Lond. 1753. oct. sect: 4. of the Effects of opium in a Diarhaea & vomiting.[13] sect: 7. in the Dysentery.[14] Heisters. Med: Chirurg: & Anatomical Obs. V.1. No.84 of the Bloody flux & Diarhaea.[15]

23. [*continuing from p. 21*]
accustomed to it; but sometime thereafter it became a universal draught at meals, and almost as much esteemed as the small English table beer, especially when drunk with a crust toasted bread and scraped Nutmeg.

[*margin:* from eating fruit, or catching cold on Duty] Some say it proceeds from eating fruite; & others from catching cold on Duty. the Distemper decreased as the fruite went out <of> Season, though the drinking of beer continued. The latter end of September & beginning of October were remarkably wet and cold, which no doubt promoted the distemper & I believe was the chief cause, especially as we came from a better quarters to a worse, and doing night Duty to which we were strangers at home[a]. The Streets here are very flat, & when the raine falls it lyes long, which makes the Streets wet. tho not dirty the feet are always wet and damp: nor are the Flemish Shoes so good as the English.

[*margin:* None of the Officers Ill of it, & only three Servants.] None of the Officers were ill of this distemper and only three of their Servants,

24. [a]none of our Spring Recruits were troubled with Grieps or purging, nor had they the Ague. they joined us when the weather was dry & warm.

25. [*continuing from p. 23*]
being less exposed to the injuries of the weather, have good dyet[x] good wine. wine and water for their common drink, good lodgings, good fire,

---

[12] John Huxham, *Observations on the Air and Epidemic Diseases from the Year MDCCXXVIII to MDCCXXXVII inclusive: Made by Dr. Huxham, at Plymouth: Together with a Short Dissertation on the Devonshire Colic*, trans. John Corham Huxham (London: J. Hinton and Henry Whitfield, 1759–67), I, xxxi. This is the translation of Huxham's *Observationes de aere et morbis epidemicis, ab anno MDCCXXVIII ad finem anni MDCCXXXVII* (London: Joannes Hinton [etc.], 1752 [vol. I first published in 1739]), I, xxiv.

[13] George Young, *A Treatise on Opium, Founded upon Practical Observations*. (London: A. Millar, 1753), sect. 4 (pp. 33–9).

[14] Ibid., sect. 7 (pp. 47–52).

[15] Heister, *Medical, Chirurgical, and Anatomical Observations*, trans. George Wirgman (London: J. Reeves [etc.], 1755), I, obs. 84 (pp. 108–9).

(Par: 5t) are warmer cloathed than the men; plenty of ripe fruits of which they eat freely, nor do they seem to be unwholesome

{"A man will pass his summers in health, who will finish his luncheon with black mulberries which he has picked from the tree before the sun is trying."}

Hor: Sat:6. lb:3. v.21.[16]

[*margin:* Ague.] Par: 8. Agues were contemporary with the above desease, & regular Quotidians.

[*margin:* Method of cure.] on the first complaint I order a Vomit about an hour befor the fit, by which it's often rendered shorter; none withstood an ounce of the Bark given in Brandy or Gin, taking a dram every two or three hours. I give the Bark to the Trooper & he puts it into his Dram bottle, without any formal preparation, taking it on Duty*. and it's a just observation of Abercromby de variatone

26. ˣSalmon in his Universal Traveller V.i p.170. fol __ observes, that those that live well, & can afford good kitchene physic in unhealthfull Countries, come off better than; the common Soldiers and poor people. it is very certain, says he, where good wine or punch, & good food are taken moderately, they contribute to preserve our healths in unwholesome Countries[;] he treats of the Diseases in India where the English escape some diseases which are common among the Natives; which some impute to providence, but he to their manner of living.[17]

*Fred. Hoffman Op.Med.Tom 3 de recto cortuis chinea usu in febribus intermittentibus.[18]

27. [*continuing from p. 25*]:
pulsus Sect. 3. **{"Prudent men considered him a preeminent doctor. He did not administer a great quantity of remedies, but only the very least that was necessary to conquer disease."}**[19] only two were obstinate and were brought from England; in which case, if the Bark failed, it was the Hospital practice to give a half a Drame crude Sal

---

16 Hor. Sat. 2.4 [not 6].21–3.

17 Thomas Salmon, *The Universal Traveller; or, A complete description of the several nations of the World* (London: R. Baldwin, 1752), I, 170. This entire passage refers particularly to India. "Those that live … unwholesome" is quoted; the remainder, paraphrased.

18 "Of the correct use of cinchona bark in intermittent fevers": Hoffmann, *Opera omnia physico-medica*, VI, cap. 5, pp. 32–41; James provides a translation in *Medical Dictionary*, under "quinquina."

19 David Abercromby, *De variatone, ac varietate pulsus observationes* (London: Samuelis Smith, 1685), p. 46.

Ammoniac, every third hour, with some bitters, such as Decoct: Febris: amar. Fuller:[20] & I have often seen it succeed.

[*margin:* Agues not cured by sudden frights.] It is a common notion that a sudden fright will cure the ague. January 14th 1743 Ashberry of Major Jenkinson's troop[21] was almost recovered of an Ague & that day sent a foraging, fell into the Scheld unexpectedly, was heartily ducked and frightened; yet the Ague returned at its usuale time more violent than formerly, & was afterwards cured by the Bark. the same happened to our Sutlers Servant,

28. **{"[Trying] a variety of remedies is the daughter of ignorance."}** Verulam[22]
{"Nothing hinders a cure so much as frequent change of medicine."} Sen. Epist. 2.[23]

29. [*continuing from p. 27*]
but instead of curing the Ague, occasioned a violent inflammatory fever. vid: Hor: Sat: III. lib:ii. V.293.[24] there are many private receipts for the cure of an Ague, and every body has his own favorite & I have been complimented with many, & it would be endless to mention them.

[*margin:* Bark the most certain remedy.] it's needless to enquire for a more certaine remedy than the Simple Barke, if the disease once form into a regular Ague, I am certaine it will cure and never saw it faile. I think it best in Substance and whatever is added only increases its bulk but not its virtue; unless it be to a very weake Stomach in order to make it sit easie. in very obstinate cases I order thus. **{"Take ½ oz. of the finest Peruvian bark, powdered, 6 gr. flowers of sal ammoniac, 3 gr. camphor and enough conserve of wormwood to make a bolus;**

---

[20] "Fuller's bitter fever decoction" was named after Thomas Fuller (1654–1734), who developed it.

[21] Charles Jenkinson entered the Blues as a cornet, 8 Nov. 1712; capt., 5 Feb. 1723; major, 10 Dec. 1739; lieut.-col., June 1745, and until his death, 21 June 1750. His son and namesake had a distinguished career as an M.P. and a major figure in several cabinets, including a tenure as Secretary at War (1778–82). WO 27/1, return for Blues dated June 1750; RADCP, Box 3/47; *Army List for 1740*, p. 6.

[22] Despite Buchanan's ascription, this quotation does not appear to come from Verulam (Sir Francis Bacon).

[23] Seneca, Epistles 2.3.

[24] "Should chance or the doctor raise the sick lad up from his peril, his crazy mother will kill him by planting him on the cold bank and bringing back his fever. What is the malady that has stricken her mind? Fear of the gods"; Hor. Sat. 2.3.293–5. *Horace: Satires, Epistles and Ars Poetica*, trans. H. Rushton Fairclough, The Loeb Classical Library (Cambridge, Mass.: Harvard Univ. Press; London: William Heinemann Ltd, 1955 [first printed 1926; revised, 1929]), p. 139.

one quarter to be taken every hour, washed down with Fuller's bitter decoction, already noted."}[;] upon recovery some of the

30. [*facing p. 29; blank*]

31. [*continuing from p. 29*]
men eat a Lemon with its skin, on such days as they expect the fit.

[*margin:* A Woman takes one ounce of Bark at a Dose.] A woman of the Regimt took an Ounce of the Bark in warm water overnight instead of a vomite, complaining of weight at Stomach next morning, & finding out the mistake, took her vomit, & brought it up. had the appearance of a slight jaundice, but soon went off, & the Ague afterwards cured by the Bark.

[*margin:* Agues local or partial.] Agues are sometimes partial or locale, seizing some particular part of the body, viz: the face or head, at a certain hour, & exactly resembling an Ague, & cured by taking the Bark, & some apply plaisters of the Bark to the part, & that with success.

[*margin:* a horse has an aguish disorder, & cured by the Bark.] I remember to have seen a horse of Captain Ramsdens[25] have an aguish disorder, & cured by the Bark, & drinking the chalybeate water of Sunninghill Well on Windsor forest.[26]

[*margin, top of p. 33:* Agues more frequent in the lower part of Ghent than in the upper.] it has been observed that part of the Garrison quartered

32. [*facing p. 31; blank*]

33. [*continuing from p. 31*]
on the high ground of St. Peter's hill in Ghent, has been less subject to this desease, than these who are in the lower part of the town & near the canals:

[*margin:* more common amongst the foot than horse.] the foot more subject to it than the horse, being more exposed to the injuries of the

---

[25] Frecheville Ramsden (b. c.1717) was commissioned a cornet in the Blues on 17 Feb. 1742; lieut., 24 July 1745; capt., 26 Feb. 1755; lieut. and lieut.-col., 1/Horse Grenadier Guards, 8 Feb. 1762; sold his commission and retired, 8 June 1768. RADCP, Box 3/47; WO 27/4, return for Blues; *AL 1756*, p. 14; *AL 1767*, p. 19; *AL 1768*, p. 19.

[26] Equine ague is described in E. R., *The Experienc'd Farrier: Or, a Compleat Treatise of Horsemanship. In Two Books; Physical and Chyrurgical.* 2nd ed., enl. (London: W. Whitwood and A. Feltham, 1691), pp. 128–9. On Sunninghill Well, see P. H. Ditchfield and William Page, eds, *The Victoria History of Berkshire* (London: St. Catherine Press, 1923), III, 134. Its water was probably intended to serve as a tonic for the horses.

weather in doing Duty, having no watch-cloaks. our Troopers have a good warm cloake & strong boots, & less duty.

[*margin:* Agues not occasioned by Spirituous liquors.] Drinking Gin & Spirituous Liquors are said to occasion this distemper; our foot Guards are remarkable for this taste, yet not much Subject to the desease, and all our drunken fellows have escaped the distemper.

[*margin:* more frequent at Bruges than at Ghent.] it was almost universal with the garrison at Bruges, especially where their barracks were moist & cold, there their arms soon rusted, belts moulded & contracted; that town is not so well inhabited as Ghent. the neighbourhood more watery, the air more damp, for want

34. [*facing p. 33; blank*]

35. [*continuing from p. 33*]
of fire. vid: Hipp: de aere, locis et aq:[27]

[*margin:* agues cured by change of air only.] As part of Bruges garrison marched thro Ghent to Germany, some soldiers had been ill of agues upwards of twenty weeks, were sent to the Hospital, where some recovered without Bark or any other febrifuge medecine, which was entirely owing to a warmer & dryer air. I have observed the same in England when our Regimt. marched into Kent or Essex to escort his Majesty, the further we marched towards the marshy grounds & the longer we stayed, Agues were the more frequent, & as we returned into Hertfordshire, some cured of themselves, especially if the weather was favorable. the same is observed by those who travele into the fens of Lincolnshire.

[*margin:* No Officer or Servant ill of the Ague.] None of the Officers have been ill of this desease, nor any of their Servants; a plain proof that the air of this Country is not the only cause of

36. [*facing p. 35; blank*]

37. [*continuing from p. 35*]
the distemper, but that it rather proceeds from the Soldiers manner of life. few of the inhabitants were ill of this or Par:7. this desease may proceed from the same causes as Par.7. for both decreased about the same time. viz: by the latter end of November, & by this time our men were more healthie; being now more habituated to the climate, have put up Grates

---

27 Hippocrates does not deal with dampness per se in "Airs, Waters, Places," but does claim that inhabitants of marshy areas are especially prone to summer quartans: *Hippocrates*, trans. W. H. S. Jones, The Loeb Classical Library (London: William Heinemann, Ltd; New York: G. P. 'Putnam's Sons, 1931), I, 85.

and keep good coale fires. Agues were common next Spring, chiefly quotidians, and cured as above.

[*margin:* an Irish cure for an ague.] Our Irish additionals attempted to cure themselves, by grating a twopenny Nutmeg, adding an equale quantity of common alum & Sugar, divided into three equal parts, taking one in a Glass Vinegar just befor the fit, but were often obliged to have to recourse to the Bark.

[*margin:* an English cure] Some of our Troopers from Essex affirm that two Drams Groundsell Seed taken in warm water or Beer an hour before the Aguesh fit begins, proves a certain cure, drinking something warm & continuing in bed to procure sweat. this I tryed, but never

38. [*facing p. 37; blank*]

39. [*continuing from p. 37*]
with Success. it always occasioned weight & Sickness at Stomach, with inclination to vomite, & never had any Sudorifick quality more than what could be occasioned from the method of keeping warm[x].

[*margin:* an Ague cured by Seasickness.] I knew an obstinate Ague cured by severe Seasickness in going from England to Holland, was four days at sea in a violent storm, vomited violently; had taken large quantities of the Bark without Success, but never had the least aguish disposition after landing.

[*margin:* my own Case.] I catched this distemper June 17th. by lying under my Markie only, having neither tent nor curtains, the weather very wet & stormy, my bedding damp, & sometimes wet; was seized every other day, the fever violent five or Six hours, with severe Shiverings, breaking out into violent sweats.

> **{"Cold sweat poured down my beleaguered limbs and the dark drops rained down from my whole body. Wherever I put my foot a pool trickled out, and from my hair fell the drops; and sooner than I can now tell the tale I was changed to a stream of water."}**
>
> Ov: met: lib: 6. V.632.[28]

as soon as the

40. B. having an obstinate Ague was advised to drink a bottle of Brandy as an infallible remedy; this plasing [*sic*] his Taste, sent immediately for a Bottle, but by mistake a Quart of Anniseed water was brought, which he finished in a few hours, got excessively drunk, had a violent fever for some days. The Ague continued & was at last cured by the Bark.

[28] Ovid, Metamorphoses 5 [not 6]. 632–6.

41. [*continuing from p. 39*]
Sweating appeared was instantly relieved; the first access of the fever was so violent that I was blooded^ <^I have blooded many Troopers in the first access, & don't think it retarded the cure.>, vomited nixt morning,

[*margin:* takes an ounce Bark dayly] took the Bark ad oz. i pr. diem in Strong Mountain white wine, dr. ii pro dose, without any visible operation; the first ounce entirely prevented the return of the fit, & the Second compleated the cure: many scabs broke out about the mouth & lips, which was common with others & certain forerunner of recovery. Nixt morning after taking an ounce of the Bark I perceived the real taste of it in my mouth, having entered the blood & tinctured the Saliva.

[*margin:* Relapse.] I relapsed July 20th tho not so violent & imagined it proceeded from catching cold on the 17th Inst. having worked hard after pitching my tent, dressing the ground, &c. sweated much. afterwards, lying upon my bed in my westcoat only, falling asleep, the walls of the tent being tucked up & a strong draught of air; took the Bark with the same success as befor, eating the slice of a Lemon in order

42. [*facing p. 41; blank*]

43. [*continuing from p. 41*]
to take off the taste.

[*margin:* The Barke is sometimes purgative.] I have heard of the purgative quality of the Barke, but never saw it prove so excepting in one case, where it purged so violently that the Gentlemen [*sic*] was obliged to give over its use; if at any time he found himself costive a small <dose> proved a gentle laxative:

[*margin:* Opiates are then to be given with it.] in this case Opiates are to be mixed with it.

[*margin:* Agues frequent when encamped in wet low ground.] During the month of August 1745 we were encamped in low[x] wet grounds on the Side of Brussells Canal, the Ditches & Pools of water full of green flax which gave a desagreeable smell, especially towards evening or after raine; the <water> could not be drunk by man or horse; had large dews & thick fogs every night; & here agues were frequent.

[*margin:* Agues not so frequent in Garrison at Antwerp as we expected.] The latter end of this Season we were in garrison at Antwerp; Agues were not so frequent as we expected from the report of the Inhabitants, probably were prevented from the dry frosty air, which continued during our short stay in garrison. <vid.> Heister's Medical,

Chirugical & anatomical obs. v.i. No. 82 of the method of curing the Ague among the Soldiers.[29]

44.

ˣSanctorius accounts for the bad effects of a moist Atmosphere. S.ii. Aph:viii. **"In a foggy Air Perspiration is lessened; the Pores are obstructed, and the Fibres weakened and not rendered more firm, and the Weight of the retained Matter is both perceivable and injurious."**[30]

45. [*continuing from p. 43*]

[*margin:* The Small pocks.] Par: 9. The small pocks were Epidemick at Ghent about the time we marched into Garrison; many of the inhabitants were seen in the Streets with very fresh marks, & some with perfect Pustules;

[*margin:* The Flemish use the cool method.] were mostly children; are treated in the cool method; the children often running about the house & seldom confined to bed; are seldom mortal, nor are they near so apprehensive of catching them as the English are.

[*margin:* & affirm they have them two or three times] and affirm that it's no extraordinary thing to have them twice or thrice, & I have been assured of the same from their Physicians. Mr. Stevenson, Surgeon to Durure's Regimt[31] assured me he attended on of his Soldiers twice for this distemper since he came to Ghent.

[*margin:* begin with us in December] Some of our troopers were seized with them in the month of December 1742 <& one officer January 26th 1743>. were of the distinct kind.

[*margin:* Method of cure.] I treat them after Sydenham's manner, only I endeavour to procure a stool every Othr day, by dyet or Clister, &

---

29 Heister had attended Dutch troops in 1708–09, and the treatment for ague that he delineates in *Medical, Chirurgical, and Anatomical Observations* (I, obs. 82 [pp. 107–8]) was associated with this time.

30 *Medicina Statica: Being the Aphorisms of Sanctorius, Translated into English with large Explanations. Wherein is given A Mechanical Account of the Animal Oeconomy, and of the Efficacy of the Non-Naturals, either in bringing about or removing its Disorders: Also with an Introduction concerning Mechanical Knowledge, and the Grounds of Certainty in Physick.* trans. and ed. John Quincy (London: William Newton, 1712), p. 136.

31 James Stevens [*sic*] served as surgeon to the 12th Foot ('Whetham's, later 'Duroure's) 20 April 1732–c.22 Nov. 1744. He then settled in Pewsey, Wilts., where he appears to have practiced until at least 1798, in his later years working in association with his son and namesake. He may well have been the James Stephens who was buried in Pewsey 12 March 1799 (private communication from Steve Hobbs, archivist, Wiltshire and Swindon Record Office). Johnston's *Roll*, p. 8 (#135); *The Medical Register For the Year 1783* (London: Joseph Johnson [1783]), p. 117; Wallis and Wallis, *Medics*, p. 569.

by so doing many bad Symptoms are prevented,[32] but would rather have it by Dyet so as to empty the

46. [*facing p. 45; blank*]

47. [*continuing from p. 45*]
whole tube of the Guts, & for this purpose I advise roasted apples, stewed pears, currant or Plumb: Gruelle, now & then a draught of whey, &c: it's well known how foetid Stools are after the body has been bound during the course of the Desease, which is often the case from the feeding on milk pottage, the favorite dyet of Nurses; & the Patient is greatly relieved if at any time he has a naturale Stool. & I even venture to give a few Drams Manna on purpose to open the body, especially if there be an oppression at breast, which is the effects of a loade of excrements rather than the Desease.

[*margin:* Acid Sharp drinks agreeable to the Patient & may be indulged.] Acid Sharp drinks are longed for <about> the latter end of the Desease & may drink freely of small Sherbet, adding a little wine so to be a pleasant cordiale. a Glass small beer with a toast is extreamly grateful & refreshing; a Physician can scarcely prescribe a draught more agreeable to his Patient. is gently laxative & promoting to Stool. Sucking China Oranges keep the mouth and throat clean, quench thirst, & keep

48. [*facing p. 47; blank*]

49. [*continuing from p. 47*]
the Stomach in good order. some Patients eat Six or eight a day.

[*margin:* our men take no great pains to prevent pitting yet escape as well as their Neighbours.] Some people are at great pains to use Oyntments, washes, &c: to prevent pitting; this is not much minded with our Troopers, yet escape as well as their neighbours; I advise them not to pick the Scabs off, but give them time to dry & fall off; sometimes wash with warm milk, <Buttermilk> or boil elder flowers in milk; their nurses often use Goose Grease. The only extraordinary covering which a Trooper has is his cloake for the first three or four days;

[*margin:* too much covering or hot rooms are dangerous.] but Gentlemen are too apt to keep themselves too warm for fear of the Desease strieking inwards. & often attended with dangerous consequence; & the bad effects of too much heat is very evident upon some of their acquaintances coming to see them. it's then common for the servant to

---

[32] Sydenham popularized the "cool" treatment of smallpox. Whenever possible, patients were to be exposed to cool, fresh air. Their diet was to be cooling, laxative, and diuretic.

help & stir up the fire, probably an extraordinarie candle or two brought into the roome, &c: I have <observed> the Patient change suddenly from being quiet & easie, become tossing & tumbling, sighing and

50. [*facing p. 49; blank*]

51. [*continuing from p. 49*]
sobbing & gasping for breath, but soon recover upon the Company going away, the room cooling, opening the curtains & moving the bed clothes; in the Hospital there was a roome appointed for the small pocks, it was small & narrow, too much crowded with beds, & an Iron Stove in the midle with Seacoale; these Stoves are soon overheated, & make a suffocating air, & I am certain one of Coll: Beake's men was actually suffocated there[a]. this distemper disappeared nixt Spring.

[*margin:* two men lye in an open Barn & do well.] Nixt July two Troopers were seized with this distemper in Camp, & removed to the neighbouring village, were distinct & favorable, lay in an open barn & had a slight flux during the whole course of the Desease; milk & water boyled with crust of bread was their common drink, adding a small quantity of brandy and a lump Sugar. Decoct: Diascord: thus prepared was their common medecine: {**"Concoct 1 oz. diascordium with a sufficient quantity of boiling water to makes 2 lbs.; stirring, add 4 oz. deflagrated spirits of French wine [i.e. brandy] and sweeten with white sugar** [continues p. 53]

52. [a]Huxham observes that the small pox in Plymouth 1740. 1741. 1745. among the Sailors, Soldiers & Prisoners had commonly the most evident Symptoms of the malignant fever with the small pox, which therefor proved exceeding fatal among them; whereas many person in the neighbourhood, that had no communication with the hospitals, & were otherwise tolerably healthy, had a very favorable kind. it's certainly of the highest ill consequence to confine such putrid air, & the sick in it. the absurd method of making a kind of hospital chamber in a house, & crowding up two, three, or more sick in it, is a most dangerous practice, and I have known it manifestly fatal. the Stench, the groans, the cries of one disturb & offend the others: its rare they sleep all together, but they are too often kept waking so; it's bad living by such Neighbours. &c: vid: Essay on the Small Pox.[33]

53. [*continuing from p. 51*]

[33] John Huxham, "An Essay on the Small-pox," *An Essay on Fevers*, introd. Saul Jarcho (Canton, Mass.: Science History Publications [Eatson Publishing Intl.], 1988; repr. of 3rd [1757] ed.), p. 70. "Among the Sailors … favorable kind" is a quotation.

to taste; 3 spoonfuls to be taken every third hour and an opium pill every night at bedtime."} both did well, living on Ryce Gruell & thin Broths.

[*margin:* The Hospital practice.] water gruell acidulated with vinegar is their common drink in the Hospital, stools promoted by Dyet or Clyster, Opiat pil at bedtime if restless: are purged as soon as they turn & blooded if the Second fever appear. we had only the above two this Campaign.

[*margin:* Women & children have them in the open field & do well.] Some of our Women & Children had them in Campaign 1745. one walking abroad dayly & doing her common business of washing, &c: till the eight [*sic*] day, not knowing what ailed her, the pustules very large & flat. lying in a cold tent on wet ground, was purged with Senna & Prunes, & keeped a whey Dyet some time. This year they were frequent in the Hospital of the confluent kind, very mortal, few recovering: many of our children had them in the open Field and did well; a whey dyet was their only physick. they were common amongst the country people in our Dutch Cantonment, the cool Regimen always used, nor are they afraid of infection; all our men

54. Heisters Medical, Chirurgical & Anatomical obs. V.i. No.45. of the method of treating the Soldiers having the smallpox, ardent fevers, bloody flux, & Agues, in the hospital of the Army.[34]

{**"I have freed the common people from the plague more than the rich, who use many medicines."**}[35]
Sanctorius – S.i.a.139.[36]

55. [*continuing from p. 53*]
escaped; some children had them & did well.

[*margin:* Some constitutions not easely affected with the small pocks.] Mrs Royston[37] had them at Antwerp & tho' ill, came by water on board our Bagage Bylanders to Williamstadt, & did well; Several

---

[34] Heister reported the observations of a British Army hospital surgeon, Thomas Wilson, who had been confronted by several epidemics in 1707. *Medical, Chirurgical, and Anatomical Observations*, I, obs. 45 (pp. 50–1).

[35] Provenance unknown.

[36] Aph. 139, sect. I (p. 34 of *Aphorismi*) reads, "*Hinc nobilium sere nemo cum remediis, plebeii vero sive iis plures sanantur*"—"Very few of the wealthier People are cured [of the Plague] by Medicines, but a great many of the poorer Sort recover without them": *Medica statica*, p. 121.

[37] Possibly a matron, nurse, or cook, although she does not appear on any list of hospital staff and servants; she may have been tied to the Horse Guards and nursed in the regimental infirmary.

Troopers were on board who never had the distemper, nor did they catch it. My Landlady at Brussells never had the small pocks. she has ten children & all have been ill of this distemper except the Youngest. She nursed all her children & lay with them during their illnes, yet never had the distemper. the Youngest is about three years of age, lay in the same cradle & bed with its Brothers & Sisters, yet never had the least sickness. I know many instances of this kind, some Physicians & apothecaries attend them dayly, & I am told never had them[a]

[*margin:* Method used to prevent infection] In England this distemper is thought very infectious, & many people avoid coming to market for fear of catching it; the common custome is to carry a Nosegay of Green Rue at which they often smell, or stuff some into the

56. [a][*crossed:* Some Constitutions are proof against infection – Sanctorius[38]]

At my Lodgings in Nottinghame, a Young Lady had the distinct small pox, & tho five people were in the same house, who never had them, none were seized with the distemper at that time.

I have often Lodged where the family never had the small pocks, & tho I attended this desease dayly it never appeared in the family.

Jany. 1750. they were Epidemick at Stafford near two Years & it was remarkable that the Apothecaries family were amongst the last who had them.

They are said to be most infectious upon change of air. 1750. a troop of Sr. John Mordaunts Dragoons came to Stafford Nov. when the Desease was common, many of the men never had them, nor were any of them taken ill; & nixt April the Regmt. was reviewed there & continued twelve days in town, yet none seized with the distemper.

Lord Aston[39] 1751. often visited at Stafford whilst the small pox was Epidemick in town & Country, but did not catch the Distemper. but was seized with <it> Augst. 1751. when it was neither in town nor Country & dyed of the Confluent sort after the turn; of an inflammation of the Lungs, to which his Lordship was naturally subject. his Brother lived to the same Age Viz. 28. & dyed of the same distemper. which has been always fatal to the family, none ever recovering [*crossed:* this distemper].

---

38 Buchanan's crossed observation recurs on *ms. p. 286*. In Quincy's translation, aph. 135, sect. I, reads, "They are soonest infected [with Plague] who have weak Lungs; they who have sound ones the contrary": *Medica statica*, p. 120 (cf. *Aphorismi*, p. 33).

39 James, 5th Lord Aston of Forfar, died at Tixall, a family seat, 24 August 1751 and, as Buchanan would be, he was buried at St. Margaret's, Stafford. *LM*, XX (1751), 428; *GM*, XXI (1751), 381.

1754. we had no small pox at Stafford but they were common at Newport & some neighbouring villages, with which we corresponded dayly. in 1755 we had them at Stafford & not in the neighbouring villages.

I knew two Mothers, nurse, & lye with their Children when ill of the small pox & neither of them catched the distemper, tho then Epidemick, but some years thereafter were taken ill of this desease & dyed.

Mrs. Clarke's Son had only one small pock on his back, large as a small boyle, & turned on the eight day; yet at first he was very sick, & it was thought he would have many. she knew the like Instance on a Girl.

57. [*continuing from p. 55*]
nostrills; many go to London where the distemper always reins. to prevent the infection of the Country, & other come from town into the country.

[*margin:* Some imagine they are caught from change of air.] others imagine they may be caught from change of air. viz: going from one place to another, yet I never observed any thing remarkable of this, unless the desease prevailed in the town as at Worcester 1737. where it greatly raged in town & Country, being chiefly confluent, was very mortal, the Summer hot & dry.

[*margin:* Some imagine themselves infected from seeing an infected person.] Some are frighted at the sight of a person lately recovered[x], & imagine themselves to be infected; go home with this notion, are unease & sicken, having complaints the same as preceeding the eruption, & should be treated in the same manner as if the pocks were at hand. & tho they do not appear at this time, & the person recover, I have seen them come soon thereafter.

[*margin:* Method used by the Nurses in England.] Common Nurses are fond of the hot method, keeping the Sick always in bed with much covering, the roome close shut up & good fire, greatly

58. a Mother catched the distemper from her child which she suckelled, when the child recovered the Mother was taken ill, & being but slightly indisposed, suckeld the Child, on its body were several large boyles resembling small pox ripened &c. 1760. the small pox in the neighbouring villages some months; & appeared at Stafford June. were Epidemick at Burton upon Trent, a Young man coming here to visite his friends broke out, & they began to spread.

[x]this I knew happen to a Butcher's Boy, who seeing a person in market with fresh marks, was suddenly surprized, went home, sickened, & broke out in a few days. a Girl seeing a woman begging in the Streets, & a child in her arms with fresh marks of the smallpox, was freightned, run home, telling her Mamma she had catched the desease from a poor

woman, & begged to give her a penny, which she did, & broke out the 3d. day.

a Servant Maid seeing another in market just recovered with fresh marks; was suddenly surprized, freighted, went home & sickened, imagined she should have them, had a violent fever & dyed the 3d. day without any eruption. N.B: she was plethorick & had an aversion to bleeding &c: many livid Spots appeared on her body after death; when first seized had the fluxus Mensis very large.

59. [*continues from p. 57*]
use the Safron bag, viz: Safron tyed in a rag, soaked in Sack, & squeezed into their common drink mixing ale with their small beer, giving a Glas Sack in order to bring them out; feeding & filling with milk pottage; apply a rasher of Salt Bacon round their throats, commonly put a red hot pocker into their beer to prevent a sore throat, endeavour to keep the body bound & costive; treacle water their favorite cordiale about the turn, & rub the face with Goosegrease. it's no rare thing to see full grown people & aged ill of this distemper.

[*margin:* in Scotland.] in Scotland the nurses use the cool Regimen, always bleed on the first complaint seldom confining to bed except the three or four first days, drinking green tea or fig tea, water gruell with currants, clystering with milk & Sugar in which a small quantity of the bark is boyled. hands & feet dayly bathed in warm milk & water, wrapping them in warm flannel; washing the mouth often with Honey of Roses, jelly of Currants & Green tea; a small list of

60. [*facing p. 59; blank*]

61. [*continuing from p. 59*]
flannel round the neck; Syr: Diacod: much used when the complaints begin. Sack whey or small Cinnamon water the chief cordiale. Manna the common purge or Syr: Rosar: cum Senna. the face nibed with Creame. it's rare to see full grown people ill of them, being almost confined to children & not near so mortal as in England.

[*margin:* few dye of the distinct sort and few recover of the confluent sort.] as it has been my constant custom to keep an exact journal of Regimental Practice, I find eighteen cases of the distinct small pocks of or belonging to the Blews, and all recovered, one was from inoculation. of the confluent sort there are Eleven cases and eight of them dye.

[*margin:* Lingring fever.] Par: 10. About the beginning of Octr. 1742. a small lingring fever appeared which engaged the attention of Physicians and Surgeons more from it's being <more> mortal than frequent. it always began with grieps & purging, pain at Stomach & bowells, tongue dry & parched, voice weak & broke, a deafnes, the eyes staring, mouth always open, looks unnatural & stupid, skin dry & burning, pulse low & frequent, a universal stupor & weakness.

{**"Like this, my booby sees nothing, hears nothing; what he himself is, whether he is or is not, he does not know as much as this."**}

Catull: ad Colon.[40]

[*interleaf, pp. 61-62*] Small pock Cases Septr. 29th. 1756.

Distinct No. 107. all recovered except one & that a sucking Child, teething, attended with looseness, Convulsions &c: I was called the day befor she dyed, the pock was favorable & came to maturity 8th. day.

Confluent No. 31 – 22 dye, – N:B: are mostly Adults.

Inoculation. No. 27 – all distinct & do well, not one in danger.

[*back of sheet*] Distinct, No. l.l.l.l. Inoculation No. l.l.l.l.l.l.l. Confluent No. l.l.l.l.l.l.

62.

Sheeps dung infused in black cherry water, is a favorite with the Nurses, in order to bring them out.

[*margin:* Yellow fever.] in Decr. 1743. we had the yellow fever, so called from the yellow colour of the Skin, & was more dangerous than frequent. the first complaints were sickness and weight at Stomach, with frequent retchings to vomite; bleeding & Emeticks were usfull; the yellow coloured appeared the 4th or 5th day.

[*margin:* Method of cure.] I then ordered Saline Saponaceous medecines with the {**"Decoction of nitre (Edinburgh recipe) and 1 oz. manna"**} [;] as the body was commonly bound. this proved sufficiently opening; there was a constant pain about the *Regio Hepatica* when pressed, & always eased by fomenting; towards the latter end of the distemper frequent vomitings were troublesome, but in some measure prevented by mixt: antemetic: nostr. these were followed with laborious breathings & other deadly Symptoms viz. hiccups, starting of the tendons, wyld looks, playing with the bed cloaths. & generally ended in death. Haven of Capt. Shipman's[41] died the tenth day:thought his illness was occasioned by the fatigue of marching

63. [*continues from p. 61*]

---

40 Catullus, Carmina 17.21–2.

41 Charles Shipman (b. c.1700) entered the Blues as a cornet 6 May 1719; capt.-lieut., 18 July 1737; capt., 25 April 1741; major, 17 Dec.1754. He retired 17 Dec. 1756 and died 15 Nov. 1767. WO 27/4, return for Blues; WO 64/11, p. 10; RADCP 3/47; *Army List for 1756*, p. 14; *GM* 563.

[*margin:* Causes.] the patients commonly complained of catching cold on Duty, perspiration seemed to be obstructed and to have fallen on the bowels. None of our drunke fellows catched <it>.

[*margin:* Method of cure] The method of cure was with Diaphoreticks, Cordials, Blisters, &c: they were seldom attended with any visible operation or good success; blisters never altering the pulse; refrigerating medecines were tryed to as little purpose; warm fomentations were at least used & seemingly with good success. pains in the bowells were eased, the tongue moistned, the skin cooled & softned; some sweated, which was promoted with Sperm: Cet & Sal: V:C.C. the stupor abated, & all things promised a cure but few recovered. few died under twenty days & many lived beyond thirty, never had a visible crisis;

[*margin:* none of our men recover.] none of our Men recovered;

[*margin:* no Officer or Servant ill of this fever.] none of the Officers or their Servants were ill of it. it decreased about the end of Janry 1743. It appeared at Bruges by the end of July. Decoct: Serpent: was their chief medecine & bleeding was thought hurtfull.

Corporal Goodyear of Sr James Chamberlaynes[42] troop was taken ill Octr 26. & sent to the Hospital

64. [*continues from p. 62*]

a foot from Germany, overheating himself & catching cold. his urine was always high coloured, having nothing like that of a jaundice, and his Stools of a naturale colour. never tasted any thing but medecines & always laye on his back. Aldridge of Cpt. Wenman's[43] of a corpulent habit of body & old Drammer, lived to the 20th day. was to all appearance in a fair way of recovery, but relapsed suddenly & dyed suddenly. Goodine of the Major's[44] was treated as the above two & recovered, tho often in great danger, & lingered for a long while & took Decoct. Serpent. many died at Ghent. Dr. [*written heavily, to obscure "Mr."*] Austine of Genl. Haley's Regmt.[45] opened one of their men & found the membrana adiposa full

---

[42] Sir James Chamberlayne, bart., entered the Blues as a cornet 2 May 1718; capt., 20 Jan. 1732; major, June 1745; lieut.-col., Nov. 1750; sold out, 17 Dec. 1754. He died in Oxfordshire 23 Dec. 1767. RADCP Box 3/47; WO 27/1, 2, 3; WO 64/11, p. 10; *Army List 1740*, p. 6; *GM*, XXXVII (1767), 611.

[43] Richard Wenman was commissioned a cornet in the Blues, 7 May 1709; lieut., 9 Sept. 1726; capt., 10 Dec. 1739. His death is noted by Buchanan below, *ms. p. 99*. WO 64/10, f. 8; *AL 1740*, p. 6

[44] Troop commanded by Charles Jenkinson (n. 21).

[45] Adam Austine (d. 1773) was surgeon to the 1st (Royal) Dns., 8 July 1742–July 1748. He received his M.D. from Glasgow in 1749—and seems to have practiced entirely in Edinburgh, being established there at least as early as 1752. Although he did not publish, he appears to have enjoyed a good reputation, and he was successively elected a member of the Royal Company of Surgeons and a fellow of the Royal College of Surgeons (and

of yellow thin liquer in the abdomen, at least a quart of the same liquor within the Peritaneum; all the viscera of the same colour. the liver in its natural state. no Stone or concrets in the Gall bladder or Ducts. the Gall bladder containing a black inspissated glutinous liquor, rather thicker than gelly. a large quantity of yellow liquor was contained in the Thorax. the liver weighed nine pounds. None of our Officers were ill of it, & it disappeared with the month of Janry.

65. [*continues from p. 63*]
Decr. 17th, was treated as above & died 27th. he had a constant hiccup which never yeilded to medicine.

[*margin:* Dissection No. 1.] I opened his body, the Peritoneum was livid & black, quite mortifyed; the Omentum much wasted & mortifyed; all the intestines black & mortifyed, & in some parts adhering strongly to each other; a strong putride smell; the Stomach inflamed and beginning to mortify. the Pylorus much inflamed, it's sides thicker than usuale & the passage very narrow, the Spleen of a whitish colour & appeared as if it had been macerated some time in warm water. the superior surface of the liver of it's naturale colour, but was hard to the touch; the exterior membrane of the large Lobe seperated from its substance, & adhering to the inside of the ribs; many large abcesses with good *pus* were found here, the whole being a mass of corruption, the Gall bladder full of deep yellow bile, much yellow water in the pericardium. all other viscera sound. N.B. during his illnes he never made any <particular> complaint about the Regio Hepatis, nor was there any Symptom of the liver being in this morbid state, nor any thing of this kind suspected by the Physicians. was a remarkable sober man.

[*margin:* No. 2.] Serjeant Clark of the Second Regmt of Foot Guards.

66. vid: an historical Dissertation concerning <the> malignant Epidemical fever of 1756. with some with some account of the malignant Diseases prevailing since the year 1752. at Kidderminster. by James Johnstone M.D. 8o. Lond. 1758.[46]

an Essay on Bilious fevers, or the history of Bilious Epidemick fever at Lausanne in the 1755. by S: A: D: Tissot M.D: Lond: 1759. 8o.[47]

Royal College of Physicians) of Edinburgh. Johnston, *Roll*, p. 13 (#245); Wallis and Wallis, *Medics*, p. 20.

[46] James Johnstone, *An historical dissertation concerning the malignant epidemical fever of 1756* (London: W. Johnston, 1758). This reference to Johnstone appears to be general, rather than to a specific point.

[47] The edition that Buchanan refers to was actually published in 1760: S. A. D. Tissot, *An Essay on Bilious Fevers; or, The History of a Bilious Epidemic Fever at Lausanne, in the Year MDCCLV* (London: D. Wilson and T. Durham).

67. [*continuing from p. 65*]
treated in the same manner as the above. about the latter end of the distemper had a constant grinding of the teeth especially in the night time & when a sleep: two days befor he dyed a constant craving for victuals[;] dyed Janry. 3rd. the body opened nixt day, all the intestines inflammed, especially the small ones, black & beginning to mortefie. the Stomach the same; they were slite open in quest of worms, but none found, tho strongly expected from *grinding of the teeth & craving appetite*. the liver more relaxed than usuale, the left lob covering part of the Spleen & adhering to it. the Gallbladder full of very thick & black bile; all other abdominal viscera sound; in the Thorax nothing remarkable only less water in the pericardium than I ever observed. part of the left lung adhering strongly to the Pleura, but never any complaint in that part.

[*margin:* No. 3.] Durham a Soldier of the same Regmt was taken ill Decr 19th & dyed Janry 22d. Stomach & intestines the same as the above; the Bile thin of a yellow brown colour. the heart very large & much Water in pericardium, a thick white membranous

68. [*facing p. 67; blank*]

69. [*continuing from p. 67*]
Substance three inches long contained in the heart, but not fixed to any part. the lungs full of blood & many black Spots on them, but no where adhering to the Pleura. N:B: this patient had always a tickling dry cough, & pectoral medecines never had any good effect. did it proceed from the largenes of the heart interrupting the motion of the Lungs? as all men have different complexions, features, make &c: nature seems to have observed the same rule with regard to the inside, for we observe great variety as to it's size form &c: hence probably different tempers, passions, &c.

[*margin:* No. 4.] Wyld of the 4th Troop of Guards dyed of this fever Janry 22d. complaints were more moderate than the above three. upon opening the body the lungs adhered strongly to the Pleura, yet never any complaints in breathing; much fat about the heart & no water in the pericardium; Stomach & intestines sound but much distended with wind; the liver sound; the Gall thin & of a brown colour; other viscera sound & naturale, only the neck of the bladder inflamed. The braine being dissected,

70. [*facing p. 70; blank*]

71. [*continuing from p. 69*]

in the right ventricle was a large abcess, containing much thin green coloured pus, insinuating itself thro the whole substance of the right hemisphere, the same found in the left hemisphere; the veins very large & turgide, in the Cerebellum was an abcess of the same nature; & pus found as the Medulla passes through the foramen & guessed about four ounces, N:B: an abcess in this braine was never suspected & must have been some time aforming; yet this person answered all questions very distinctly, had no involuntary motions till the day befor death. viz: his face convulsed.[48]

[*margin:* Experiments on the Gall] The following experiments were made on his Gall. Viz

Expt 1st. Some Gall was dropt into common vinegar, sunk to the bottom & coagulated, growing so tough as to be lifted up with my probe. there was no effervescence.

Expt. 2d. when juice of Lemon was dropt on a small quantity of the Gall, it was the same as in expt 1st.

Expt. 3d. Oyle of vitriol being dropt on the gall it coagulated presently, was harder than in 1st & 2d, white; no effervescence.

72. [*facing p. 71; blank*]

73. [*continuing from p. 71*]

Expt 4th. Ol: Vitriol being diluted with water, & mixing some Gall, it sunk to bottom, coagulated, but not so hard as in expt. 3d. of a mixed colour of white & green resembling liquid Soape.

Expt 5th[.] Gall being mixed with Spt. C.C. did not effervesce, nor coagulate, nor change colour.

Expt. 6th. Ol. Rosar. diluted in water, & adding some Gall, when gently stirred with my Probe, there was a regular mixture & remained as a liquid Soape, no change of colour. vid: Pag. 62.[49]

[*margin:* Inflammatory fevers] Par: 11th. Inflammatory fevers were neither Frequent nor dangerous during the winter 1742.

[*margin:* Method of cure. Bleeding.] my method of treating them is bleeding largely vizt: an lb: i. if the pulse be full & strong, youthfull or sanguine constitution, & sometimes requires to be repeated; (frequent sighings with oppression at breast, indicate bleedings, as frequent reachings indicate Vomits). If any sickness at Stomach, mouth & tongue clammy, with reachings to vomit; vomiting is absolutely necessary. I commonly use Ipecacoan:. Some people have a certain prejudice against vomites.

---

48 An autopsy, almost certainly 'Wyld's, is discussed in Francis Home, *Medical Facts and Experiments* (London: A. Millar; Edinburgh: A. Kincaid and J. Bell, 1759), pp. 11–13. Home alludes to "the surgeon," in all probability Buchanan.

49 Which work "Pag. 62" refers to is unclear.

[*margin:* warm water a good vomite.] I then order them to drink two or three quarts warm water in order to wash the Stomach, &

74. [*facing beginning of section on inflammatory fevers*]
Heister's Medical, Chirurgical & Anatomical Obs. V:i. No. 81. of the cure of Inflammatory fevers among the Soldiers &c.[50]
{"I commence the Cure of all acute Fevers, by letting Blood."}
Bagl: Prax: Med.[51]

75. [*continuing from p. 73*]
often provides a good emetick: let the patient be never so sick, he is easely perswaded to drink warm water when freightened at the name of a vomite. its operation is mild, promoting sweat & urine, especially when assisted by an opiate which is my common practice, & seldom fails of procuring a good night, & gentle sweating, especially as the humours have been well diluted by the warm water & moved by the shoake of vomiting. I order them to bed so soon as the vomite is over, take the opiate, drinking something warm, viz: Negus or small punch, & this often surpasses expectation.

{"But medicines drunk for these fevers are capable of acting in such a way that the body remains in its accustomed state of heat and coolness, not abnormally heated nor abnormally chilled."}

Hipp. de affect.[52]

[*margin:* Sicknes at Stomach:] if Sicknes at Stomach yet continues & there be reason to think it is overcharged from overeating; which is often the case: it's then necessary to repeat the vomite, in order to bring up its contents[a];

[*margin:* require two or three vomits] but our men don't care to have it repeated a second time tho' absolutely necessary. I then make them up in different forms, writing

76. [a] **{"Unless the vessel is clean, whatever you pour in turns sour."}**

---

[50] Heister, *Medical, Chirurgical, and Anatomical Observations*, I, obs. 81 (pp. 106–7).

[51] Giorgio Baglivi, *The Practice of Physick, 'Reduc'd to the Ancient Way of Observations. Containing a Just Parallel between The Wisdom and Experience of the Ancients, and The 'Hypothesis's of Modern Physicians. Intermixed With many Practical Remarks upon most Distempers* (London: Andrew Bell [etc.], 1704), I, cap. xiii, p. 166 [p. 120 in Baglivi, *De praxi medica ad priscam observandi rationem revocanda. Libri duo. Accedunt dissertationes novae* (Leiden: Fredericum Haringium, 1700)]. Buchanan may have quoted the passage in the text from Johnstone, who likewise quoted it (*Historical Dissertation*, p. 55) without specifying chapter or page; cf. below, n. 322.

[52] Hippocrates, Affections, 18.

Hor: Ep.ii. lib:1.[53]

77. [*continuing from p. 75*]
the Stomatick, Cordiale &c:

[*margin:* method of giving them.] advising them to drink warm water if squeamish or sick, at Stomach. vid: Hor: Sat:iii. lib:ii. V.145.[54] Vomits are the most universal operation, & being so much used are almost despised; one or two are thought sufficient for any desease, but are not near sufficient in gross habits & foul feeders.

[c] {**"But whatever other pains, because of summer heat, afflict the breast and heart, administer lukewarm water with a small amount of honey and a hemina [about 1 ½ pints] of vinegar added and, after a short time, if the illness continues, [the patient] should vomit, being kept free from heat and clothing; but, if after vomiting the pains oppress him again and suffocate him, I provoke another vomit or purge with much warm water."**}

Hipp: de affect:[55]

[*margin:* Troopers love to be worked heartely.] Troopers love to be worked heartely, & so much the better if it operates upwards & downwards, & seldom blame a strong vomite but will always find fault with a weake one. I seldom exceed dr. fs. Ipecac: or gr. vi Tartar. advising a Glass wine after the operation.

{**"In cardiac disease the one hope of relief lies undoubtedly in wine."**}

Plin: lib: xxii.[56]

I prefer Ipecacoan to Tartar, tho I cannot say I ever saw any bad effects from Tartar providing they drink freely, but if they

78. [c] {**"Not only in the Beginning, but in any Stage of the Disease, the Stomach is to be washed out, if there is an Urging to vomit, or if there is a bilious, foetid, and very disagreeable Eructation."**}

Huxham. de Aere et morb: Epidemic: Lond. 1752. V.2. p.48.

---

[53] Horace, Epistles 1.2.54.

[54] Hor. Sat. 2.3.145–50 reads (*Horace* [trans. Fairclough], p. 165): "Now once [Opimius, a miser] fell into a lethargy so deep that already his heir was running in joy and triumph round about his keys and coffers. But his physician, a man of very quick wit and a loyal friend, revives him by this device. He has a table brought in and bags of coin poured out, and bids many draw near to count it."

[55] Hippocrates, Affections, c.15.

[56] Pliny, Natural History, 23.25.50; cf. below, n. 388.

vid: Cels: lib:i.C.3.[57]

79. [*continuing from p. 77*]
do not, some remains & sticks to the coates of the Stomach & occasion violent sicknes some time thereafter, as was the case with Smith of Capt. Wenman's, was extreamely sick with violent cramps, involuntary stools, convulsive motions in the Stomach, but cured by drinking freely of warm water & oyle, & then a large opiate. it's seldom prescribed in this country. The morning after the vomite they often find themselves much better, being more *lightsome* as they express it. I then enquire into the state of their body, whether they go to stool or if their belly feel full, which if it does, purging is necessary;

[*margin:* purging medecines necessary.] pil: cocc: minr: answer the intention, but if the case require a sudden operation, then Sal: cathartic: amar: with Manna, or Pulv: Jalap: worked off with water gruel or warm small beer, do the business, & op: h:s:. Infusion of Senna with prunes is a common medecine, drinking a cupfull every hour till it purges. Some object against purging medecines, saying, there is nothing in them to work upon, having eat nothing these three days. we see dayly good effects from a vomite, tho the water come up as

80. [*facing p. 79; blank*]

81. [*continuing from p. 79*]
clear as when drunk; great advantages may be obtained from purgative medicines tho the Stools are not excrementitious, there being a large discharge from the Glands of the Gutts. so in a cold the head is greatly relieved by a large discharge of clear thin water thro the nostrills, though no snot passes.

[*margin:* Droughts.] Drought is a constant attendant of fevers & very troublesom to the Patient.

{"If no amount of water could quench your thirst, you would tell your story to the doctor."}

Hor: Ep.ii. lib:ii V:146.[58]

---

[57] Huxham, *Observations on the Air and Epidemical Diseases*, II, 69 [Latin quotation in Huxham, *Observationes de aere et morbis epidemicis*, II, 48]. Huxham himself quoted Celsus 1.3.[20]. The passage in Celsus to which Buchanan refers is probably this: "When ... there are bitter eructations, with pain and weight over the heart, recourse should at once be had to a vomit"; De Med. 1.3.20; cf. Celsus, *De Medicina*, trans. W. G. Spencer, The Loeb Classical Library (Cambridge, Mass.: Harvard Univ. Press; London: William Heinemann Ltd, 1960 [1935]), I, 61.

[58] Horace, Epistles, 2.2.146–7.

Our men commonly drink Sage tea from the universal custom of England, to which I add the Squeeze of a Lemon or Ora<n>ge and Sal: Prunel: oz. i. to each quart; is a pleasant & gently sudorifick especially if a little wine be added which is necessary as a Cordiale.

[*margin:* Acid sharp drinks often wished so may be indulged.] Acid sharp drinks are often [*crossed:* are often] wished for, & I know none so pleasant as the common sherbet made rich with fruite, of this the sick seldome tyres, tho he soon dislikes all other drinks; a little brandy or wine[x] may be safely added to take off the <u>waterishnes</u> as the men phrase it, is then a real cordiale, & good diluter.[59] Peppmt.

82. [x] **{"The nearer a Fever approaches to the height, the less we insist upon**
refrigerating Remedies, for fear of opposing the Crisis."}
Bagliv: Prax: Med: lib:i. C.13.[60]

83. [*continuing from p. 81*]
water is very agreable. Decoct: Nitros: P:E: is an excellent medecine & a neat form: if the body be costive sweaten with Manna instead of sugar. Sal Prunel is the most universal medecine in this case, mixed in all drinks or given in powders, is one of the best febrifuges. Negus is a favourite drink with our men of which they drink freely with Spt. Nitr: Dulc: gt. xxx. in each draught[;] having a pleasant smell, it's extreamely agreable to the Sick; holding tamarinds in the mouth or sucking oranges greatly quenches thirst; the mouth should be often washed with common drink in order to relax the Glands; all drinks to be drunk moderately warm & freely. nature demands it.

[59] Wine was the most common and esteemed cordial. Dilutents, which included such thin liquids as water, whey, ptisans, and juleps, were intended to thin the blood when it was viscid. Ptisans were a staple of Hippocratic medicine. Boerhaave, who believed that inflammation was caused by stagnant, thick blood, recommended that the condition be combated by having the patient drink some thin, watery, hot liquid, in order to dilute the stagnating bodies. Rollo reported that in the practice that he had observed in the West Indies, when intermittents were in the cold stage, liquids were not provided to the patients, but that as sweating approached, "free dilution was recommended, as lemonade, toast and water, barleywater, &c." John Barker, *An Essay on the Agreement betwixt Ancient and Modern Physicians: Or a Comparison Between the Practice of Hippocrates, Galen, / Sydenham, and Boerhaave, in Acute Diseases. Intended to Shew, What the Practice of Physick, in such Distempers, ought to be* (London: G. Hawkins, 1747), pp. 103–5; Herman Boerhaave, *'Boerhaave's Aphorisms: Concerning the Knowledge and Cure of Diseases*, 3rd ed. (London: W. Innys [etc.], 1755), pp. 98–9 (aphorisms #398–400); Dancer, *Brief History of the Recent Expedition*, p. 56; Quincy, *Lexicon PhysicoMedicum* (1719), p. 115; Rollo, *Observations on the Diseases on St. Lucia*, p. 74.

[60] Baglivi, *Practice of Physick*, I, 167; cf. *De praxi medica*, I, cap. xiii, p. 122.

[*margin:* Sweating.] Fevers often attempt to throw themselves off thro the Pores of the skin, breaking out in sweats, & if naturale, are of great service & often compleat the cure. when I perceive a naturale inclination to sweat I encourage it by drinking freely of the above drinks, encreasing the quantity of wine & covering warm, which ought to be done with prudence for fear of encreasing the fever.

[*margin:* Sudorific Medecines.] Lap: contrayerva

84. [*facing p. 83; blank*]

85. [*continuing from p. 83*] is much mixed in their drink or given in powder. I commonly use Ther:Androm:& a few grains Camphire[x] & a large draught small warm punch & generally succeeds well, & is keep't up by drinking plentefully; water gruell sharpened with vinegar is an excellent medecine at this time; if skin feel hot & burning, parched and dry, warm, bathing would be the best medecine, but we have no conveniency for it.

[*margin:* to be used with caution.] One should be cautious of forcing sweats at this time; the body should be washed with a spunge in warm water, especially under the arm pits, Groins &c: soaking the palms of the hands in warm water, as also the feet; coming out of the sweat, care should be taken to dry the body well, have fresh linnen &c.

[*margin:* the men have their own favorite medecines.] The men deal much in hot pots for this purpose; or treacle posset, boyled beer or buttered ale; & no <bad> medecines if they are not made too strong. in slight complaints it's their common custome to drink a pint cold water, when going into bed. The Officers use Sack whey & Spt. C.C. seldom exceeding a tea Spoonfull which is too small a Dose.

86. [x]Fred: Hoffmanni Op: Med: Tom:3. de Camphorae usu interno securissim et preestantissimo.[61]

87. [*continuing from p. 85*]

[*margin:* Headach.] Fevers are often attended with violent headachs, the patient complaining his head is so heavie that he cannot raise it from the pillow; often giddy as a Goose, like to tumble down, & if he stoops to buckle his shoe, cannot get up again. face is flushed eyes bloodshot, eye lashes heavie, can hardly be kept open; the above method greatly contribute to remove it. but applications should be made to the part affected. the nose is commonly stuffed up & dry, with weight or pain about the eyebrows; the head is greatly relieved if you can make the Nose run.

---

[61] "On how to use camphor internally most safely and with the best results;" Hoffmann, *Opera omnia physico-medica*, VI, pt. 1, pp. 60–7.

[*margin:* Method of cure.] I order them to hold their heads above the steam of warm water or sage tea, Sucking the vapour thro the mouth & drawing thro the nostrills; there's a large discharge from the nostrills, Corners of the eyes & glands of the mouth, & often times much clotted blood from the Nose, as was the case of Cornet Ramsden's Servt., to the instant relief of the Patient; & should be repeated two or three times a day; taking care to keep warm & prevent

88. [*facing p. 87; blank*]

89. [*continuing from p. 87*]
catching cold. the men at first despised this simple method & when advised to bath their feet at bedtime in order to ease their head, used to laugh at it, as a childish thing, but seeing its good effects, became a common practice amongst them. Leeches may be applyed to the temples & seldom faile of giving ease; if the headach yet continues with inclination to dose & sleep, Blisters are absolutely necessary to the nape of the neck or behind the Ears, & should be keept open till all complaints cease; the only inconveniency of attending them is the Strangury, for which I order marshmallow tea, or dissolve Gum Arabic in their common drink.

{**"Whenever headaches occur, the head should be warmed by washing it with much hot water, and sneezing should be encouraged to carry off phlegm and mucus."**} Hip. de affect:[62]

{**"Then the head in general [should be treated] but vapor-baths through the ears and nostrils .... One should avoid sun, wind, fire, smoke, and sharp-smelling substances. He should live quietly and enjoy a mild diet; his lower belly be thoroughly emptied."**} de Morb: lib: iii: Hipp.[63]

90. [*facing p. 89; blank*]

91. [*continuing from p. 89*]
[*margin:* Dyet.] The Dyet can hardly be too simple. I recommend that as in the small pocks, Par: 9. I often consult the appetite & seldom forbid what the Patient wishes for, unless it be something very much out of the way[C]; there's a natural aversion in all sorts of fleshes, but thin broths with toasted bread are proper, boyled turneps, &c: Sparrowgrass, &c:. what I commonly order is the crumb of a penny loafe boyled in a quart water over a gentle fire into a pint, adding a Gill wine when near boyled; seasoning with Cinnamon, Nutmeg Cloves, sweatning with

---

62 Hippocrates, Affections, c.2.

63 Hippocrates, Diseases III, c.2.

Sugar; makes a good nourishment, & real cordial, easely got & easely prepared. Our men on recovering their appetite are apt to indulge too much & return to their gross way of feeding befor the Stomach be strong enough to digest it; <{**"With difficulty will you be kept, when hungry, from the appointed feast."**} Ov: rem: Am: V:631.[64]> become sick at Stomach & relapse. must begin again with Vomits &c.[a] Puddings they think to be light food & may eate freely, but theirs are made of flower & eggs, boyled very hard, & become a tough paste, not to be dissolved by a weak Stomach; light

92. [c] {**"One should humor some patients as it were, so that they have food and drink provided cleanly and whatever the patient feels or touches should be pleasant. For others they should not be exposed to great harm, or only that which can easily be remedied, such as cold while there is need. With these it is advantageous for the doctor to be agreeable to the patient, regarding what he talks about, his appearance, his clothes, his haircut, his fingernails and his smell."**} Hip: de morb: vulg: lib:vi. S:vii.[65]

[a] {**"When one consumes more foods or drinks than he is used to, or of a different kind, it is best for him to immediately vomit them up."**} Hip: de affect:[66]

93.

bread puddings may be allowed. & small fish viz. Pearch, Gudgeons, smelts, Plaise, &c: with little butter & seasoned with Salt & lemon[a]:

> {**"Fish, both boiled and baked, alone and together with other foods, are light food."**} **Hip: de affect:**[67]
>
> {**"If you wish to give something restorative, to assist recovery, give spelt or a wheat ptisan .... The weak should then receive food; then give them generous wine .... Prepare and give to the weak common food and main dishes that will not cause flatulence, belching, acid, or colic, and will cause neither looseness nor constipation. The weak should receive light food that will not trouble the belly or the body by heat or bloating, or fulness, but be quickly digested and passed through the stomach."**} Ib.[68]

---

64 Ovid, Cure for Love, 631.
65 Hippocrates, Epidemics, VI.iv.7.
66 Hippocrates, Affections, c.61.
67 Ibid., c.52.
68 Ibid., c.44, 46, 47.

{**"If fever persists, give broth of meal or millet; if foods are given, only small amounts should be provided, together with laxative main dishes."**} Hip: de intern: affect:[69]

{**"After this, however, give pure foods for lunch, meals to provide strength, and [the patient] should also drink wine."**} Ib.[70]

{**"And then there is diet too; that I may perform all a physician's part, I will tell you what to take and what to shun."**}

Ov: Rem:Am: v.795.[71]

94. [a]a regular dyet is the greatest consequence in Recovery, but much neglected from our unsettled way of life; & works surprizing changes both on man & beast, of which I have an extraordinary Instance; having kept a Young fox, even in the field, & feeding him daily with boyled or roasted meats, he became very tame & tractable; as he was a great favorite with all the Regimt, the <men> would sometimes treat him privately with a Young-live-Rabbite, or pigeon, or give him some warm blood; nixt day he was wild as ever, and would not suffer himself to be handled, tho at other times he might be played with as a young-puppy, & required a carefull diet some days, befor he returned to his mild & gentle temper.

{**"So, when wild beasts have lost the habit of the woods and grown tame in a narrow prison, they lose their grim aspect and learn to submit to man; but, if a drop of blood finds its way to their thirsty mouths, their rage and fury return, and their throats, reminded of their old life by the taste of blood, swell again; their anger boils up and scarcely spares their frightened trainer."**}

Lucan: lib:4.[72]

95. [*continuing from p. 93*]

[*margin:* Regimen:] The Same Regimen to be observed as in Par: 9. The patient not be always confined to bed, but suffered to sit up & let the bed cool; he had better rest himself upon the bed, than be always confined in it. nor am I too scrupulous in forbidding Company.

[*margin:* Recovery] in order to recover strength, a light nourishing dyet is necessary, & a Glass wine viz. a Gill pr. Day.

---

69 Hippocrates, Internal Affections, c.1.

70 Ibid.

71 Ovid, Cure for Love, v.795–6.

72 Lucan, 4.237–42.

{**"Wines that are sweet, dry, honeyed, and aged are the most laxative. They provoke the most urine and nourish. And they do not cause flatulence, colic or fullness .... For the body is warmed by the wine, and this heat causes the body to expel the food and drink and similar things."**} Hipp: de affect:[73]

[*margin:* many relapse from error in dyet:] Elixr. Vitriol, is proper to whet the appetite, but they should be careful not to overheat, but in this they exceed dayly, Adams of Captn. Marcham's[74] had almost killed himself by eating too freely of a bullocks heart & afterwards drinking near a quart strong Spanish Mountaine[a].

{**"By ham and by sausages rather does [appetite] crave to be pricked and freshened. Nay, it would prefer any viands brought smoking hot from untidy cookshops."**}

Hor. Sat:4 lib.2. V.60.[75]

{**"Whatever he gained, he gave to his greedy maw."**}

H. Ep.15: lib:1. V.32.[76]

I never

96. [a] {**"When food is consumed in excess of what nature can stand, disease is caused, as the treatment shows"**} Hip: Aph. No.17. S.ii.[77]

Fred: Hoffmanni Op: Med: Tom: 5. p.283. de Convalescentiae Statu, eiusque impedimentis
et Praendiis[78]

97. [*continuing from p. 95*]
allow above a pint of wine in 24 hours. If any slight feverish chilness or shiverings remain, the Bark in Substance or in tincture & taken in wine, removes it.

[*margin:* Rieding (*sic*) of great service.] I order the Trooper to ride his horse so soon as his Strength permitts; it's needless to purge them afterwards with strong physick, for that keeps them long weake; but it's of service to keep the body laxative, & our Stomatick pills answer this purpose, taking two or three as occasions require, using gentle exercise.

---

73 Hippocrates, Affections, c.48, 61.

74 Thomas Marcham or Markham became a cornet in the Blues 26 Feb. 1712; capt.-lieut., 7 Jan. 1733; capt., 18 July 1737, until his death, 4 Sept. 1755. RADCP, 3/47; *Army List for 1740*, p. 6; *GM*, XXV (1755), 428.

75 Horace, Satires, 2.4.60–2.

76 Horace, Epistles, 1.15.32.

77 Hip. Aphorisms, 2.17.

78 Hoffmann, *Opera omnia physico-medica*, V, 283, does not accord with the topic that Buchanan cites.

{"At first, let [the patient] take only short walks, so that he is not fatigued .... [Let him] exert himself a little at first, then a little more, but never very much"} Hip: de intern: affect.[79]

[*margin:* many complaints from bad Nursing.] many complaine of not being well nursed; when they have an appetite, & victuals not ready at that time, the appetite is lost again; as we have no regular nurses the sick are nursed by their Comrades, & it cannot be expected that they are so carefull in giving their medecines, as they ought to be.

{"The art of being timely is almost a medicine: wine timely given helps, untimely, harms."}
Ov: rem: Amo: V:131:[80]

98. [*facing p. 97; blank*]

99. [*continuing from p. 97*]
when the Stomach is very weake I order a large draught whey with cons: Ros: every morning: & have seen weake people recover strength wonderfully, & ascribe their recovery to this simple remedy, more than to all the Drugs they took.

[*margin:* Critical days.] I have no great regard for criticale days. by the above treatment this fever terminated in five or Six days, but may be continued longer by a different method; this was the most common fever during the winter & all did well, none being so bad as to require the Hospital.

[*margin:* Urine seldom inspected. rather trusting the looks, voice, & breathing than pulse or urine.] I seldom examine the Troopers urine, they having no proper conveniency to keep it, and think I can form a better judgement from their voice, looks & breathing, than from their pulse or Urine[a]. Capt. Gaye's pulse intermitts every third stroake even in a good state of health. Capt. Wenman died the 16th day Pleuretick & asthmatick; his pulse & urine were always more favorable than his look & breathing.

{"Forestus writes that in the Delphic plague ... some people had an excellent pulse and yet died; Galen also asserts this."} vid: Diemerbroeck de pest. p:21. 103. et[c][81]

100.

[a] Majr. Jenkinson in the white of the left eye has a bloody Specke & when it encreases in bulke & Spreads large, it's an undoubted Sign that his

---

[79] Hippocrates, Internal Affections, c.1.

[80] Ovid, Cure for Love, v.131–2.

[81] This passage is actually a quotation, from Ysbrand van Diemerbroeck, *Tractatus copiosissimus de peste* (Geneva, 1721), I, cap. vii, pp. 26–7.

body is then Plethoricke, requires bleeding. otherwise he is soon purcy & choaked up at breast, is then suddenly seized with a pain in the left cheeke & Gum. face swells especially from catching cold, any slight debauch. & then bleeding & purging are necessary. this is a family distemper, his Sister is often affected in the same manner, & applies a Leech to the Gum. he was formerly subject to dangerous inflammations of the Lungs, Spitting blood &c: from which he has been free Some years, & thinks it changed to that in his face. when his tent is damp & wet, he is sure to be troubled with whizzing coughs & bad breathing, but recovers in dry weather.

101. [*continuing from p. 99*]
et Car: Piso Obs: Med: p. 222x.[82] Tulpis: Obs: p. 257[83]

{"In the French, the arterial pulse is quicker and freer. In the Germans, it wavers and falters. In the Belgians, it is more sluggish. In the English and Scots, it is much fuller and stronger .... Otherwise, in any place you please under the sky, the pulse of the veins quivers [as among] those who live in mountains, open plains, mountain valleys or forested places."} Abercromby de variatione ac varietate Pulsus[84]

{"Nevertheless, you may discover many teachers of the art of Apollo who, when they visit the sick, handle their pulses according to their custom, not from skill but handling in a comical way."} Ib: Lectori[C.].[85]

[*margin:* Causes.] The principal cause of this fever is cold; all complaining they catch cold on Duty, patrolling the Streets in the night time, putting on a damp Shirts [*sic*], lying in damp sheets, being wet aforaging &c: few or none acknowledging their own private debauches. & such as have been sometime in the hole[86] are sure of it, with aching pains in the bones & cured by plentifull sweating[a.]

---

[82] On p. 222 (sect. iii, cap. iv) of *Selectiorum observationum et consiliorum*, noviss. ed. (Leiden.: Cornelii Boutestein and Joh. Arnoldum, 1714), Charles le Pois [Carolus Piso, d. 1633] asserts that in recognizing fevers associated with asthma neither the pulse nor urine is a good indicator. Instead, he advises that diagnosis of these fevers be confirmed by the presence of heat, internal and external, and of such accidental signs as lassitude, oppression at the breast, watchfulness, and thirst.

[83] Nicolaas Tulp, *Observationes medicae*, 6th ed. (Leiden: Georgium Wishoff, 1739), cap. xlix, pp. 356–7. Tulp (d. 1674) asserts that some pulses naturally intermit; laymen may become frightened on noting any intermission and this may bring on imaginary illness.

[84] Abercromby, *De variatone pulsus*, p. 8.

[85] Ibid., p. 9.

[86] The hole was a detention facility for soldiers who had committed minor crimes or infractions.

[*margin:* Pleuretick fever.] Par: 12th. Pleuretick fevers did not appear till Decr 1742

102.

[C] {**"The sick person should have times of conversation also, and of quiet, and he should say what he may wish, and his conversation should be considered, whether he is loud or says a lot and whether what he says is true or false."**} Hip: de morb: vulg: lib:vi. S:vii.[87]

{**"Also note the state of his mind and intellect, how it is in itself, apart from any medical treatment and anything foreign, whether he tends to be sad or joyful, fearful or confident, hopeful or despairing."**} Ib.[88]

{**"The body should also be considered: sight, hearing, touch, smell, tongue, and reasoning."**} Ib.[89]

vid: Cels: lib: iii. Cap:vi {**"For the pulse upon which we mostly rely is a very deceptive thing, because often it is rendered slower or faster by age and by sex and by constitution"**}[x].[90]

[a] fevers of this sort were frequent after coming into Garrison 1743. seldom lasting above 6. or 7. days, were not dangerous excepting to hard drinkers & several dyed; they drank too freely with their old pot-companions, talking of our German expedition &c. and seldom complained till it was too late. vid: Fred: Hoffmanni Op: Med: Tom: i. p.84. Lect.1. Cap.xi. de febribus Petechialibus veris.[91] et Ibid. Cap.x. de febribus Epidemicis, Exanthematicis, Catarrhalibus sive Petechirantibus[92]

103. [*continuing from p. 101*]

and encreased towards Spring, they attack suddenly & there's no time to be lost in attempting a cure.

{**"When winter fevers arise […] one must take care and be observant."**}

Hipp: de affect:[93]

& Horace well advises

---

[87] Hippocrates, Epidemics VI, 8.7.

[88] Ibid., 8.10.

[89] Ibid., VI, 8.17.

[90] Celsus, De Medicina, 3.6.5.

[91] "Of true petechial fevers," *Opera omnia physico-medica*, I, sect. i, ch. xi, pp. 84–93; cf. *System of the Practice of Medicine*, I, 167–82.

[92] "Of fevers [called] epidemic, exanthematous, catarrhal, or even petechial." *Opera omnia physico-medica*, I, sect. i, ch. 10 (vol. II, pp. 75–84); cf. *System of the Practice of Medicine*, I, 154–66.

[93] Hippocrates, Affections, c.12.

{"If your chest or reins are assailed by a sharp disease, seek a remedy for the disease."}

Ep:vi. lib:i.[94]

& in Sat:vi. lib:ii. V:147.

{"His physician, a man of very quick wit and a loyal friend."}[95]

is now of the greatest use, & as Ovid advises rem: Amor: V:81.

{"Crush, while they are yet new, the baneful seeds of sudden disease."}[96]

[*margin:* Method of cure] the general method of treating the above fever will answer the intention here;

[*margin:* Bleeding the chief remedy] bleeding is the chief remedy, & at first I bleed the patient till he is almost ready to faint, & sometimes fill a small punch bowell as I did with Cpt. Migelt[97] at Nottingham during the hard frost; sometimes stopping the orifice with my thumb, then letting it bleed afresh, & repeating it as the case requires.

[*margin:* fomenting the part.] fomenting the part & rubbing with Ungt. Dialth: ol: recent &c. it's a prevailing custom with the men to apply to the part a bag of hot oats heated in

104. [*facing p. 103; blank*]

105. [*continuing from p. 103*]

the frying pan, or a bag salt, or Scalded bran;

{"And when pain is present, warming materials should be applied."} Hip. de affect:[98]

[*margin:* Saponaceous & pectoral medecines.] Saponaceous medecines are of great service, pectorals usefull, those of the shops, viz: Dect: pectoral has many ingredients in proportion to the water & when boyled is too thick, should rather be prepared by infusion, is apt to pale the Stomach; in all Sicknesses it should be the principale care of a physician to preserve the Stomach in good order. for when that failes, adieu to all remedies, & it is often spoiled by drugs rather than the distemper. I order the men Bran-tea, viz: taking a handfull of bran on which they power a quart or two of boyling water, adding a few

---

94 Horace, Epistles, 1.6.28–9.

95 Horace, Satires, 2.3.147.

96 Ovid, Cure for Love, v. 81.

97 Henry Migelt or Miget was commissioned a cornet in the Blues 12 May 1726; lieut., 18 July 1737; capt.-lieut., 18 Feb. 1745; capt., 12 Aug. 1752, dying in this rank on or shortly before 24 April 1755. He was one of three officers in the Blues listed as wounded in returns after Fontenoy. WO 64/10, f. 8; WO 64/11, p. 10; RADCP, Box 3/47; *City and Court Register 1746*, p. 146; *AL 1754*, p. 16.

98 Hippocrates, Affections, c.10.

figs or raisings [*sic*] or slyced Liquorice; this makes a pleasant drink & good pectoral, quenching thirst when sharpened with juice of Lemon or Orange. they often drink Lintseed Tea sweetened with sugar candy, as a remedy for the cough. in the night time have a little Juic: Liquorit: in their

106. [*facing p. 105; blank*]

107. [*continuing from p. 105*]

mouth to prevent the tickling cough & keep the throat moist. this is one of the best pectorals. it's only fault is that of being too common, & therefor by some despised.-- <or Trochis: Bech: Nigr.>

{**"There is much that it befits men not to know; most of your doings would offend, did you not hide them within."**}

Ov. Art: Amat. lib:iii. V:229.[99]

infus: hispanic: Fuller: is an excellent medecine; all oyly & greasy medecines spoile the Stomach, should be gently acidulated and used with prudence. Lac. Ammon: with Oxymel Scillitic: of great service in promoting expectoration.

{**"But in order that sputum and pus may be brought upwards from the lung, give medicinal drinks by which the lung is moistened and pus cleaned upwards"**} Hip: de affect.[100]

{**"Moreover, one ought to clean the cavity** [i.e., gastro-intestinal tract] **downwards by giving a purging and cooling enema .... Administer also drinks and broth. And acidulated drinks should be given quickly, in order that the sputum from the side will be cleaned through the upper parts. When the pus begins to be cleared, bring the material lying against the chest wall to maturity by warming the side from the outside."**} Ib:[101]

[*margin:* Blisters.] A Blister applied to the part often removes

108. [*facing p. 107; blank*]

109. [*continuing from p. 107*]

the Stich; & when applyed without forewarning the patient there are no great complaints; but if You mention a blister, he will plead an excuse, saying he is yet not so bad & beg to put it off till to morrow. if You tell him of a plaister to the part he is well pleased & applies it with pleasure, nor are his complaints troublesome. I have blistered a Trooper for Sciatic complaints, has mounted Guard & discharged his Duty, without much pain; but in pleuretick cases one day's delay may cost the patient's life.

---

99 Ovid, Art of Love, 3.229–30.

100 Hippocrates, Affections, c.9.

101 Ibid., c.7.

{"But (to make the point once and for all) opportune moments in the art [of medicine] are many and varied, just as are the diseases and conditions and their treatments .... These opportunities demand haste, and a little later does not suffice, for a little later most patients die."} Hip: de morb:[102]

{"Resist beginnings; too late is the medicine prepared, when the disease has gained strength by long delay. Ay, and make haste, nor wait on the coming hours; he who is not ready to-day will be even less so to-morrow."}

Ov. rem: Amor: V:91.[103]

all the men recovered excepting one, viz: Christmas of Cpt. Wenman's, an old Drammer & gross habit of body, & dyed

110. [*facing p. 109; blank*]

111. [*continuing from p. 109*]

the ninth day. his blood extreamely siezy & green coloured.

{"This disease generally arises from drinking."} Hip: de affect:[104] –

he never could be brought to expectorate –

{"If within this period [i.e., 7th-14th day of illness] the pus is purged away from the side and expelled through sputum, [the patient] recovers; but if little is expectorated ... the disease drags on long."} Ib.[105]–

I'm perswaded this disease is often prevented by bleeding largely at the beginning & keeping a proper Regimen, & the complaints are so violent as to oblige the men to complain on the first attack –

{"Ardent fever, inflammation of the lungs, angina, inflammation of the uvula, and pain in the side [i.e. pleurisy] reach their crises quickly."} Hip: de morb:[106] –

{"These are called 'acute', and occur most frequently and violently in winter."} de affect[107]

{"From this disease, few escape."} Ib: de morbi lib:ii[108] –

Nixt Spring we marched to Brussels arrived there Febry 27th O:S: & quartered in Barracks rather better than at Ghent, being all inhabited

---

102 Hippocrates, Diseases. I, c.5.

103 Ovid, Cure for Love, v.91–4.

104 Hippocrates, Affections, c.7.

105 Ibid.

106 Hippocrates, Diseases, I, c.3.

107 Hippocrates, Affections, 6.

108 Hippocrates, Diseases, II, 46.

houses with good fires or stoves; the men cook'd for themselves as at Ghent. were no sooner arrived when

112. [*facing p. 111; blank*]

113. [*continuing from p. 111*]

[*margin:* Slight pleuretick fevers 1743.] many men, some Officers & Servants complained of colds, stiches about the breast cough, violent headach, eyes bloodshot, pulse quick; required large bleeding & gentle purging, &c : taking {**our pectoral pill with Fuller's Spanish Infusion.**} Some naturally inclined to sweat which was promoted with Ther: Androm: & Sal: V:C:C. as they recovered Scabs broke out about the mouth, lips & nose;

[*margin:* were very common tho not dangerous.] this was very common tho not dangerous, all our men recovering in five or six days.

[*margin:* four Officers taken ill in one night & two nixt morning.] four of our officers were taken ill in one night, & two nixt morning. few of our women & children escaped the distemper & all recovered. Senna tea was their common medicine; it run over the whole garrison.

[*margin:* was common with the inhabitants.] it was common with the inhabitants, especially amongst children, generally going thro the whole family, and called <u>la fievre catarrhale</u>; bleeding & pulv: Pleuretic: of the town's dispensatory was their universal medicine.

[*margin*: was Epidemick & universal.] was Epidemick all over Europe by accounts from News-papers. Dr. Pringle was then at Aix la Chapelle with Lord

114. [*facing p. 113; blank*]

115. [*continuing from p. 113*]

Stair, wrote a short account of it in that place, begging the same from me; says of the few Officers there, he had more Patients than when at Ghent with that numerous Garrison, or could have had, had he been the only Physician: calls them colds in the shape of coughs, stiches & slight inflammations, with a sort of half feverishnes. had himself for a Patient & blamed at first the sunk Situation & Sulphurous air. I imagined it was greatly promoted amongst our men from their being quartered in publick houses, the Beer much better than at Ghent, cheap & good measure, & they indulg'd pretty freely, sitting much by the Stoves, we had pleasent Sunshine weather, yet the air was cold, mornings frosty & winds N:E: the Officers dress more & change cloaths oftner than in last quarters & therefor more subject to catch cold, the ramparts are very pleasant & evening walks were frequent. had it not appeared Epidemical & universal, both

116. [*facing p. 115; blank*]

117. [*continuing from p. 115*]
Dr Pringle & I would have remained satisfied with our own private theory.
[*margin:* fever with Eruptions.] Par: 13th. Slight fevers with a slight rash on the Skin appeared about the beginning of Janry 1743. resembling bug-bites, continued three or four days, going off without any dangerous Symptoms. were treated in the cool Regimen & scarcely required medecines.
[*margin:* Method of Cure.] if the fever threatned to be too high at first it was necessary to bleed; the men continued in bed with their usuale covering only, drinking warm-<small>-punch with Lap: Contrayerv: to promote a breathing sweat. when the Eruptions disappeared were purged with infus: Senn &c:
[*margin:* neither common nor dangerous.] this was not common, nor dangerous, all recovering.
[*margin:* more frequent in Spring 1744.] It was more common in spring of 1744. & with some Physicians bleeding was much in vogue, in a few days the Patient lost 60, 70, 80, 90, Ounces, which was attended with bad success for few recovered. I seldom blooded unless difficult

118. [*facing p. 117; blank*]

119. [*continuing from p. 117*]
breathing or Stich &c: forced me, & all my men did well; a gentle sweat was always good. the Patient often blooded at the nose a small quantity about the latter end of the Desease, the blood very thin. When the pulse sinks from bleeding too freely its not easely raised by medicines.
[*margin:* & nixt Campn] this was frequent nixt Campn & treated in the same manner & same success tho in the field, all did well excepting one woman who had it to a great degree her whole body of a deep scarlet colour, lay in a cold damp tent, being wet weather, & instead of drinking something warm, would take nothing but cold green tea. dyed the 3d day Augst. 28th.
[*margin:* & in Spring 1745.] this was common in Spring 1745 tho not dangerous & the same method succeeded.
[*margin:* Rheumatick fevers.] Par: 14th. Fevers with Rheumatick complaints were frequent but neither dangerous, nor difficult to cure. the common method of treating fevers in general answered

120. [*facing p. 119; blank*]

121. [*continuing from p. 119*]
the intention.

[*margin:* Method of Cure.] if Rheumatick complaints continued Bol: nostr: ad Rheumatis: always removed them being repeated some nights with proper Regimen. The men use Mountaine flax seed infused in boyling water, drinking a cup or two till it purges. proves a rough purge & is often successfull. fomenting the part & rubbing with Lint: Volatil: nostr. covering with flannel or fur of Hare or Rabbite. a Spoonfull of Mustard seed bruised & taken in a Spoonfull of warm water at different times, was a good medecine. all did well, none required the hospital, nor were they tedeous of cure;

[*margin:* Cause.] all blamed cold as the first cause.

[*margin:* Quinsies] Par: 15th. Quinsies were frequent but not dangerous, & treated as the above fevers.

[*margin:* Method of Cure.] on the first complaint I bleed largely, even though the pulse be not feverish. wash the mouth often with warm broath or fig tea.

> **{"Then boil down figs in water, pour off the water, grind sumac [Hippocrates may have intended corn-poppies], and heat a little of this in the fig-juice; if [the patient] is able, he should gargle, but if not,**

122. [*facing p. 121; blank*]

123. [*continuing from p. 121*]

> **wash his mouth."**} Hip: de morb: lib: ii.[109]

I always use pulv. ad extrahend. Salivam nostr. in order to make them slabber & it's surprizing the great quantity of Spittle discharged from the Glands of the mouth. if the Glands of the fauces appear very red & seemengly inflammed, I make small incisions with the point of my Bistouri in order to make them bleed, to the immedeate relief of the Patient & prevent a suppuration, & sometimes apply Leeches externally[a]. observing the good effects of Blister in the pleuretick Stich, I apply one to the throat, & seldom failed of Success. if the Uvula be relaxed gargle with Brandy & Vinegar or Aq: Alum:

> **{"But if the throat becomes inflamed and swollen, give gargles .... But if the gums or any of the parts beneath the tongue swell up, use medicine that can be chewed .... If the swollen uvula hangs down and causes suffocation ... at once give gargles."**}
> Hip: de Affect:[110]

Troopers wifes often apply a warm

---

[109] Ibid., c.28.

[110] Hippocrates, Affections, c.4.

124.
[a]the parotide Glands often swell from colds. I endeavour to disperse them by Ungt. Mercurial. keeping warm with flannel, the men do not desire they should suppurate: are afraid of Scars in these parts.

125. [*continuing from p. 123*]
Dishcloath to the Throat, & sometimes a hot loafe.

> {**"But on the lower part of the neck and jaws place a cataplasm made from warm flour boiled in wine and oil, and still warm, and apply warm bread."**} Hipp: de morb: Lib: ii.[111]

putting the warm Stocking round the throat at bedtime is an old Scotch cure. they were very frequent in the Spring, & treated as above. this is one of the most common Camp deseases & the following is a favourite medecine with many. {**Take 2 scr. powdered guaiacum gum and ½ gr. elderberry rob, to make a bolus taken at bedtime.**} some make it up with Theriac: Androm: –

> {**"Put a cupping-glass on it. Soak a sponge in warm water, and apply it against the neck and jaws .... To drink give dilute melicrat, which moistens the mouth; make the patient drink barley-water."**} Hip: de morb: lib:ii.[112]

[*margin:* Coughs.] Par: 16th. Coughs were frequent & treated with Pectorals as in Par: 12th.

[*margin:* Method of Cure:] Bals: Sulphur: Anisat: was the most universal & great favourite with the men. to which I often added a small quantity Laud: & is a good medicine in old habituale

126. [*facing p. 125; blank*]

127. [*continuing from p. 125*]
coughs. Ol: Lini is much esteemed by some but is often so rancid & smells so strong that few Stomachs can bear it, unless it be fresh drawn. the best common sweat Oyle is often preferable to it. water Gruelle sweatned with honey is the best Supper & an excellent remedy. private Receipts are common, & the following is a favorite with our Men. {**Take 2 oz. each of conserve of red roses and pulp of Majorcan raisins with 40 drops of anisated balsam of sulfur. Mix capsules M.N.M. [*moles nucis moschate*; i.e. in the size of a nutmeg], to be taken at bedtime.**} Trochis c: Bech: nigr: I often substitute in place of Succ: Liquirit: which is so commonly known that it scarcely passes as medecine.

[*margin:* one of the most common deseases & often incurable.] This is one of the most common Deseases & most difficult to cure in

---

111 Hippocrates, Diseases, II, c.28.

112 Ibid., c.27.

many cases. & people are surprized we cannot cure a cold for which every body has his own favorite medecine, but dissection often Shows them to be incurable. Joyener of captn Wenman's was always subject to cough & pain at breast, & his Captn. wondered I could not cure him, for he was seldom relieved

128. [*facing p. 127; blank*]

129. [*continuing from p. 127*]
by medecine. of a florid complexion, could hardly walk being presently out of wind from the least exercise, was naturally sober & greatly Hypochondriack. was taken suddenly ill Feby 17th 1744. with laborious breathing, pulse quick, ghastly countenance; eyes fixed & senseless, knew none of his Comrades & could not speake. stools & urine involuntary. was blooded and blistered to no purpose, continued till nixt day & dyed about Noon.

[*margin:* Dissection No. 1.] I had the curiosity to open the body, the left lung was entirely useless, nothing remaining but a membranous Substance; thick & strongly adhering to the Pleura, could not be inflated. the right lung was large & in some parts adhering to the Pleura & Diaphrame, inflammed, the blood very thick & black, neither tubercles or ulcers. the heart large & much water in pericardium, very red coloured: in the right Ventricle a large Polypus, bigger than a common Walnut, when washed was white & firm, of a tough Substance

130. [*facing p. 129; blank*]

131. [*continuing from p. 129*]
resembling a common Ligament. the same Substance was found in the pulmonary Artery about eight Inches long; & in the ascending Aorta was one of the same colour & substance; many other pieces of the same substance in other blood vessells^{x}. the Spleen large & weighing three pounds & half, & some don't weigh above four ounces.

[*margin:* No.2.] a Polypus of the same nature was found in Wells of the King's Troop.[113] he dyed suddenly; was always subject to a cough & seldom relieved by medecine; of a fine florid complexion & purcy on the least motion.

[*margin:* No. 3.] Aranthrow's left lung adhered strongly to the Pleura & was perfectly Schirrus, some parts gristly & could not be extended by blowing air, & adhered so strongly to the Spine that it could

[113] The troop commanded by the captain-lieutenant of the Blues—at this time, Henry Miget (n. 97)—was known as the "'King's Troop." Arthur, *Story of the Household Cavalry*, II, 418n.

not be seperated without tearing the Substance. the upper part of the right lung adhered to Pleura & Spine, was become Schirrous & gristly*. this man dyed suddenly & a Polypus suspected, but no such thing found. all the viscera sound.

132. [x]Vid. Pechlini obs: Med: lib:ii. No.1.[114] – Fred: Hoffmanni Op: Med: Tom: 3. p.277. de subita morte et morbis aliis in sana bilibus, ex vitali Sanguinis per Polypos intercepto circuitu ortis prudenter praecavendis[115] –Ibid: Tom: 3. de usu Anatomes in praxi Medica[116] – Tom:6. p.321.de praecavenda Polyporum generatione.[117]

---

[114] Johann Nicolaus Pechlin, *Observationum physico-medicarum libri tres, quibus accessit, Ephemeris vulveris thoracici & in eam commentarius* (Hamburgi: Libraria Schultziana, 1691), II, obs. i, 201–3 ("polypus cordis veris" ["genuine heart polyp"]). Pechlin notes while great authorities such as Tulp, Bartholinus, and Malpighi, have no doubt that heart polyps exist, Theodor Kerckring disagrees and has imputed error to those who thought differently, but Pechlin wishes to defend the authority of the distinguished men that Kerckring has disparaged. [For the notes on this and the other chapters in Pechlin referred to by Buchanan (nn. 133, 464, 456), I wish to thank Darrel Amundsen.]

[115] "Of the prevention of sudden death and other incurable disorders, from an interruption of circulation or the blood by polyps." Hoffmann, *Opera omnia physico-medica*, III, cap. x, pp. 277–84; cf. *System of the Practice of Medicine*, II, 324–8. According to Hoffmann, the most common cause of sudden death, as revealed by dissection, were fibrous concretions or "polyps" that clogged blood vessels. Their presence might be diagnosed on the basis of: difficulty in breathing without apparent cause; fixed pain in the heart; frequent palpitations and anxieties from slight causes like exercise; frequent fainting; or irregular pulse. A sign of predisposition to polyps, if not their existence, was that blood drawn in venesection and injected into warm water concreted into white gelatinous filaments. Polyps could not be cured, but might be prevented or contained.

[116] "Of the use of anatomy in the practice of medicine." *Opera omnia physico-medica*, VI, pt. 2, cap. 5, pp. 124–34; translated in James, Robert. *A Medicinal Dictionary; Including Physic, Surgery, Anatomy, Chymistry, and Botany. In all their Branches relative to Medicine. Together with a History of Drugs; An Account of thir Various Preparations, Combinations, and Uses; And An Introductory Preface, tracing the Progress of Physic, and explaining the Theories which have principally prevail'd in all Ages of the World* (London: T. Osborne, 1743–45), under "anatome." Hoffmann encourages a sense of anatomy that incorporates not only the identity of each part but its function and association with every other. He regards the importance of anatomy to surgery to be generally accepted but criticizes the Stahlians (without naming them) for ignoring anatomy on the grounds that the body is merely a passive agent of the soul.

[117] "On guarding the growth of polypus." Hoffmann does not provide a chapter or gloss with this heading, and the page reference given by Buchanan does not check out. In Hoffmann's chapter on polyps and sudden death (cf. n. 115), however, he advises that the principal strategy in preventing the growth of polyps lay in diluting or thinning thick blood and in reducing the overall plethora.

*{**"[The art of healing is restricted and contained within fixed limits.] And this is no ground for finding fault either with the physician or his Art; for he pretends not to create, but to aid and assist the body, labouring with infirmities."**} Russell de Oeconomia Naturae in morb: Acut et Chron: Glandularum. Lond:1759. p.149.[118]

133. [*continuing from p. 131*]

[*margin:* Jaundice.] Par: 17th. The Jaundice appeared in Decr. 1742. was neither dangerous or frequent.

[*margin:* Method of cure] bleeding, vomiting, purging are necessary, pil: cocc: with calomel much in use, & pil: Stomatic: nostr. No.2. or 3. twice a day. washed down with tinct: Amar: & continued some days always succeeded. the Decoction of Artichoake leaves in common water or small beer, is by some esteemed a specific in this disorder, but I never had occasion to use <it>. all our men did well; none of the Officers had it.

[*margin:* was frequent in Garrison 1744.] it was frequent in Garrison 1744. were cured with pil: Stomat: nostr. & drinking Senna tea &c: tinct. Myrrh: & aloes was a useful medecine, taking 30 or 40 drops in a Glas wine two or three times a day. was never attended with any fever or dangerous Symptom. three men were ill in one roome, for which they could not give any particular reason, having messed with their comrades. probably from too gross feeding & little exercise; the men are apt to indulge too much on coming into garrison

134. [*facing p. 133; blank*]

135. [*continuing from p. 133*]

as it were to make up for the fatigue of the field.

[*margin:* seldom or never happens in the field.] this disease seldom or never happens in the field; & in Garrison I order all the jaundiced men to ride dayly, & that the most rough trotting horse.

[*margin:* nor is it frequent amongst the Flemish.] it's hardly known amongst the towns people. Dr. Van Belengen [119] has seen but one these four years, they eat very little meat, living much on vegetables. all our men recover'd dayly on marching. a melancholy sedentary life is natural in this distemper and of bad consequence if the Patient indulge it, as was

---

[118] Richard Russell, *The Oeconomy of Nature in Acute and Chronical Diseases of the Glands* (London: J. and J. Rivington, 1755), p. 150 [Buchanan's citation of the Latin original is correct: Russell, *Oeconomia naturae in morbis acutis et chronicis glandularum* (London, 1755 [not 1759]), p. 149].

[119] Unidentified. Hawkins notes that while the army was in Brussels he "was acquainted here with Dr. Van Bellingen an Ingenious Physitian": "Hawkins Journal," f. 21v.

the case with Weaver of Captn. Wenman's, being fond of an old woman's company would not stirr abroad & use exercise, I was obliged to send him to the Hospital in order to get rid of her, & tho this be a bad place for melancholick constitutions, yet he recovered with the same medecines.

[*margin:* Bark is said to occasion the jaundice.] Some blame the Bark occasioning this Desease if long persisted in. I have had some complaints of this kind, but from my own

136. [*facing p. 135; blank*]

137. [*continuing from p. 135*]
practice never had occasion to persist so long in its use as to observe any bad consequence from it. & I knew a child take scr. fs. dayly for three years, & never had the least appearance of a jaundice.

[*margin:* Gravelish Complaints.] Par: 18th. Gravelish complaints are common and Salts of Manna or Bol: Laxans nostr. with Marshmallow tea is the common method. the body should always be kept open. diluting thin drinks are of great Service viz: Green tea sweatned with honey, whey, &c: Spirituous are too forcing & of bad consequence. Onions boyled & roasted are much esteemed. the Men often use ol Tereb: in Gin, which is too hot occasioning bloody urine. Small Stones are often passed, after much pain & bloody urine, & that without the help of medecines. Brisby of Coll: Beake's passed fifteen on his march from England. having taken bol. lax: nostr. he passed one large as a horse bean, had great pain & bloody urine, saying the bolus did him a deal of good, searching his bladder & moving the Stone from Side to Side. a foot Soldier of Blyth's Regt. was sent from Bruges to the Hospital at Brussells to be cut for

138. [*facing p. 137; blank*]

139. [*continuing from p. 137*]
the Stone March 1744. of a robust constitution & about thirty years of age; endeavouring to sound him could not introduce the Catheter, there being an obstruction about the neck of the bladder. by introducing a finger into the <u>Anus</u> perceived the bladder thicker than usual. his urine had a large purulent sediment, with many small philms swimming therein, of a strong smell & always <much> difficulty in making water; dyed some days thereafter of a common fever.

[*margin:* Dissection No. 1.] On desecting the body there was a large abcess near the neck of the Bladder externally, the part hard & swelled, the bladder much thicker than usuale being almost callous, & much contracted; containing a flat Stone weighing dr.x, almost as big as half a Crown, light in proportion to its bulk, of a brownish colour, & some part covered with a Nucleus. the right kidney entirely wasted, only a thick membranous Substance remaining, containing some pus. The last rib but one of that side had been fractured. the callus very large & pointing inwards, which had probably destroyed the kidney. the left kidney was very large, being three times bigger than usual;

140. [*facing p. 139; blank*]

141. [*continuing from p. 139*]
the peritoneum adhering strongly to it & very thick; the kidney full of small abcesses, containing much purulent pus & some in the pelvis. this urether & all the blood vessels of a prodigious size, no stony concrets in kidney or Gall bladder. the carnell columnes in the heart were cartilaginous & white coloured. Saponaceous pills and lime water is a favourite with some[x]: such as are subject to gravelish complaints are always worse from drinking the strong brown Faro Beer, but better from the small white beer which is soft & Diuretick.

{**"Clean the belly a little with thyme or scammony root, and give the same drinks drunk by those suffering from strangury. While pain continues, warm especially the place where the pain is; wash with much warm water. For drink, provide boiled meal gruel infused with honey, and for diet otherwise, the patient should eat what purges most. He should drink white Mendaean wine mixed with honey or another very sweet white wine. This disease seldom goes away.**} Hipp: de affect: intern:[120]

142. Stafford 1753. a Scotch-Hollander [i.e. "Highlander"] had a confirmed Stone which was plainly discovered by sounding[.] I recommended him to the Hospital at Shrewsberry to be cut, but soon after admission he was seized with a lingring fever & dyed in a few weeks. the Surgeon performed the operation on the dead body & found the Stone so strongly adhering to the bladder that it was impossible to extract it without pulling out the Bladder. it was of a brown colour & flat; weighed one Ounce & Six Drams.

[x]vid: Whyte on Lime water. 8o. Edin. 1752.[121]

143. [*continuing from p. 141*]
[*margin:* Costiveness.] Par: 19th. Costiveness is common amongst [*crossed:* amongst] us, often proceeding from a naturale dry habite of

---

[120] Hippocrates, Internal Affections, c.16.

[121] In sect. x of *An Essay on the Virtues of Lime-Water in the Cure of the Stone* (Edinburgh, 1752), Robert Whytt reports on experiments in which he used lime water, mixed with soap or soap lees, to reduce the stone.

body; living much on Salt or smoked meats, drinking too freely Spirituous Liquors.

[*margin:* Method of Cure.] my first attempt is to make a clear passage by laxative Ptisans of Senna, Manna &c: assisted with Clysters. viz: Enema commune nostr. drinking water gruel sweetned with honey, Barley gruell with Currants &c: the best preservative against a relapse is to eat a toaste soaked in oyle for supper, live on fat broths, use exercise, there being nothing worse than Study or a Sedentary life. such as are of this constitution should be regular in going to stool dayly[x], <[x]Pechlin: obs: med: lib:3. No.12.[122]> not giving the excrements time to harden, should sit over the steam of warm water & not press too hard for fear of procedentia Ani[a].[123]

{**"To remain healthy, one should daily excrete yesterday's feces downwards."**} Hip: de morb: lib:4. vid: lib: 3.[124]

eating cheese too freely is an unwholesome dyet especially for children, as was the case with Jack Hobson

144. {**"Your anus is cleaner than a salt cellar nor do you defecate more than ten times a year."**}[125]

[a]{**"Take lettuces and take aperient mallows, for you have the appearance, Phoebus, of one straining at stool."**}

Mart: Ep.89. lib:iii[126]

{**"Take plums wrinkled by shrivelling old age abroad: they are used to lighten the load of an obstinate stomach."**}

Ib. Ep.29 lib:13.[127]

145. [*continuing from p. 143*]

after being costive nine days from living only on Dutch cheese, many hard black excrements were brought away resembling buttons[x]. by persisting in the above method naturale excrements were brought away, being often bathed in warm water. yet dyed the 12th day. was remarkably

---

122 In *Observationum physico-medicarum*, III, cap. xii (pp. 417–20), Pechlin discusses "Phantasia in corporis excretionibus moderandis" ("The faculty of imagination in managing the excretions of the body").

123 Prolapse of the bowel through the anus.

124 Despite Buchanan's reference, this quotation does not appear to come from Diseases, IV. In referring to bk. III, Buchanan may be general, as cleansing the body downwards is noted as a part of the regimen for several diseases.

125 This is from Catullus. Buchanan leaves the quotation a fragment and appears to have smudged it purposely. He then gives a fuller version on p. 146 (cf. n. 128), but omits the first line.

126 Martial, Epigrams, 3.89.

127 Ibid., 13.29.

Sprightly, but from bad example has learned to drink Drams. was often Drunk & it was thought his inside was burnt up.

[*margin:* tobacco Clysters succeed when other means faile.] never used Quicksilver or leaden bullets, & have seen Tobacco Clysters succeed when all other means failed. Dumbar of Col. Beake's troop had been costive some days on our march to Germany & greatly fatigued being carried on the baggage waggon, had taken medicines at mouth & Clysteres injected, but no excrements passed, had violent racking pains in bowells, but never any inclination to stool. as we passed at Aix la Chapelle were told these waters were a sovereign remedy in this disorder, & halting in that neighbourhood I went with him to the Bath. advising with the Physicians of that place, he was ordered a laxative Ptisane & the water to be injected as Clyster every fourth hour, to be bathed

146. :[x] {**"You do not defecate more than ten times in a year and then it is harder than beans or pebbles. If you rubbed it in your hands you wouldn't even dirty your fingers."**}

Catul. Carmin 20.[128]

147. [*continuing from p. 145*]
twice a day, drinking the water, &c: was four days in this manner & in danger of dying, but presently relieved by Clyster of Tobacco smoake.

{**"But if he cannot accept an enema, affix a tube to the mouth of a small wine skin, inflate it, and blow much air into into the stomach and intestines; when they are distended, remove the tube and immediately insert an enema."**} Hip: de affect:[129]

{**"From both the inside and the outside one should moisten [the patient]; wash him with much warm water and have him drink potions that will move the belly and evacuate urine, and give an infusion underneath [i.e. an enema], if he will accept it."**}[130]

[*margin:* Aix la chapelle Bath.] May 17th 1743, I went into this warm Bath & continued about 1/4 <hour>. I had been much fatigued by walking in boots, the day being very warm; upon bathing was greatly refreshed as from sound sleep.

{**"This is what repairs the strength and renews the wearied limbs."**}

Ov: in Epis: Heroid: No:4. V:89.[131]

---

128 Catullus, Carmina, 23.21–3.
129 Hippocrates, Affections, c.21.
130 Ibid., c.21.
131 Ovid, Heroides, 4.90.

I inclined to sweat afterwards, but did not encourage it being obliged to march in the evening. the water was warmer than new milked milk, of a milkish colour, strong sulphureous taste & smell. some say it's warm enough to harden an egg in qtr. hour, is gently purgative, Diuretick & Diaphoretick,

148. [*facing p. 147; blank*]

149. [*continuing from p. 147*]
famous for skin diseases, aching pains, Rheumatisms & Gout &c:

> **{"Its sulphur baths ... so famous for driving a lingering disorder from the sinews."}**
>
> Hor: Ep.15. lib:i. V.6.[132]

[*margin:* Dropsy.] Par: 20th. Dropsies were seldom known amongst us, tho there were some in the Hospital.

[*margin:* seldom or never cured.] the common method of cure attempted, but never succeeded, & I never saw a real Dropsy cured tho it may be palliated by medecines, tapping &c. [*penciled line in margin next to this case*] Captn. Gay was the only Dropsical constitution in the Blews, under which he had laboured some time; so soon as we returned from Germany was remarkably bad. was formerly carefull in taking dayly exercise a horseback, but since coming into Garrison at Brussels is more sedentary, only indulging in town Diversions &c: forgetting Horace's advise.

> **{"To save your own life, won't you wake up? Nay, just as, if you won't take up running in health, you'll have to do it when dropsical."}**
>
> Epist:2d. lib:i:[133]
>
> **{"By indulgence the dreadful dropsy grows apace, nor can the sufferer banish thirst, unless the cause of the malady has first departed from the veins and the watery languor from the pale body."}**
>
> Od:2 lib:2. V:13.[134]

being put on a proper course of medecines with horse exercise,

150. [*facing beginning of Par. 20.*]
a Lunatick friend of mine has been ill of a deep jaundice for some time & far gone in a Dropsy, his belly legs & thighs greatly swelled, he is dayly drunk & chiefly with Gin or double distilled aniseed water. I advised his friends to remove him from town & board him with an honest farmer,

---

132 Horace, Epistles, 1.15.6–7.

133 Ibid., 1.2.33–4.

134 Horace, Odes, 2.2.13–16.

forbidding all manner of Spirituos Liquors, & allowing only a certaine quantity of ale, from this method with the assistance of a few Hydragogue purges he recovered, & continues well

151. [*continuing from p. 149*]
found himself less purcy, but legs swelled always towards the night, & belly increased with hardness about the Regio Hypochondriaca: mercurials & saponaeceous were tryed but without success, complaints encreasing dayly, became weake & low Spirited & jaundiced-look, thighs began to swell, went for England nixt Spring, hoping a cure from his ordinary Physicians, & being some time under their care, without any relief, began to despair & be peevish in his temper.

({**"Quarrel with my faithful physicians, and angrily ask my friends [why they are eager to rescue me from fatal lethargy]"**}) Hor: Ep.8. lib:i.[135]

then put himself under Dr. Ward's[136] care to as little purpose. his method was daily sweating twixt warm Blankets. about the beginning of winter was obliged to be tapped; four Gallons & ½ were drawn off. he dyed Decr. from being a bulkie man was reduced to a meer skeleton.

{**"And finally, in place of living blood, clear water flows through her weakened veins and nothing is left that you can touch"**}

Ov: met: lib.v V:435.[137]

Succ: Porr: is greatly esteemed by the Flemish; was given to Murray of the 3: Regmt. of Guards, but had no visible operation or good effect, nor had any other medecines any good success.

152. [*facing p. 151; blank*]

153. [*continuing from p. 151*]
[*margin:* Dissection No.1.] upon opening the body, the viscera appeared as in other Hydropicks; the liver swelled to an immense bulk, containing much water & upwards of three pints real pus, & so large that the pus was taken out <in> a pint porringer. extending itself upwards as far as the 3d. rib, pushing the Diaphragme along with it & forcing the lung almost under the clavicle; the lung much wasted & of no use; the 5t & 6t. ribs carious. all the others were soft; the left lung naturale, but much water contained. was about 30. years of age & always sober. was ill

135 Horace, Epistles, 1.8.9.

136 The reference is probably to Joshua Ward, the quack doctor who operated a hospital in London. Ward developed a number of successful patent medicines, the most important of them being Ward's Pill and Ward's Drop, two popular antimonials.

137 Ovid, Metamorphoses, 5.436–7.

about Six months & always in the Hospital. the following is a favourite Hydragogue with some. {**Take 3 gr. tartar emetic and 3 oz. of the best manna dissolved in 10 oz. of common water. Two spoonfuls to be taken every 2 hours until the bowels move.**}

[*margin:* No.2.] One of Duruer's[138] was tapd & dying nixt day. the Liver was of a white colour as if pare-boiled, & so schirrus as to be almost gristly, cutting hard to the knife: the Spleen very large of a dark brown colour. & so dry as to be ready to moulder into dust, a large quantity of Water in the Abdomen. had a perpetual drought & drank much.

{**"While he seeks to slake his thirst another thirst springs up."**}
Ov: Met: lib:iii V.415[139]

{**"Nor by drinking is their thirst quenched so long as life remains."**}
Ib: lib: vii. v:566[140]

154. [*facing p. 153; blank*]

155. [*continuing from p. 153*]

[*margin:* No. 3.] a Serjeant of Cope's Dragoones[141] being some weeks in the Hospital for an Anasarca, & heated in the common method, {**for example, take 2 oz. of syrup of buckthorn and ½ dr. tartar emetic and mix with 10 oz. common water; 2 spoonfuls to be taken every 2 hours until the bowels move**} was ordered to eat Garlick, mustard Rhadishes &c. legs were scarified & much water discharged. dyed suddenly Apoplectick. upon being blooded his blood was waterish & thin. All the Bowells were sound, no water in abdomen; the Gall bladder much distended & full of Green coloured Bile, Omentum much wasted; no water in the thorax, contrary to expectation, for some imagined he had been suffocated by water in the breast. & very little in pericardium. the lungs full of blood & no adhesion, the braine quite sound. no inflammation, & not above a Spoonfull of water in the left ventricle, yet some said his death must be from water in the braine. he was of very large size as were all the Bowels, excepting the Spleen.

{**"A regimen of food and drink should be instituted, along with exertion and exercises that will restore a slim, dry physique, with very healthy flesh ....**

---

138 Buchanan may have received this information from James Stevens, surgeon to Durore's; cf. n. 31.

139 Ovid, Metamorphoses, 3.415.

140 Ibid., 7.569.

141 7th Dns. Francis Home was surgeon to the regiment 18 March 1742–Nov. 1750 and may well have been Buchanan's source on this case. Johnston's *Roll*, p. 13 (#235).

156. [*facing p. 155; blank*]

157. [*following on from p. 155*]

In diseases linked to dryness], it is best to take food only once a day, not to eat and drink to satiety, to work these off by exertion and walks, and to sleep as little as possible."} Hipp: de affect:[142]

[*margin:* Goute.] Par: 21st. The Gout is not so common in this Country as in England & our Gouty Officers are more healthy here than at home. Captain Gilbert[143] seldom escapes a fitt every fall of the leafe, but had not the least gouty complaint till Janry. 23rd. 1743. O:S: & was then occasioned by spraining the anckle.

[*margin:* Method of cure.] his method of cure is living Sparingly, abstaining from meats & strong Liquors:

{**"Does your heroic virtue and spirit defy rich suppers?"**}
Hor: Sat 7. lib:2.[144]

green tea & skimmed milk his principale Dyet, condemns the vulgar practice of strong cordials[a]. tho when in health he eats and drinks heartely.

({**"You will be loved in Rome till your youth leave you."**} Hor: Ep.)[145]

wrapps the part in flannel & keeps warm, seldome goes into bed, rather sits in his great chair, his legs hanging down, saying the humours then fall more easely downwards, the parts swell sooner, becoming numbed as it were, & pain ceases. when the swelling decreases

158. [*facing p. 157; blank*]

159. [*continuing from p. 157*]

he takes three purges, {**Equal amounts of the sacred tincture and the elixir of health, a small quantity.**} this fit was much shorter than used to be, but more painfull, which he always bears with great patience.

({**"Believe him brave and good."**} Hor[146])

he had a slight fit nixt <month of> March & only held for four days. is often Subject to bleeding piells, which were stop'ed some time, but

---

[142] Hippocrates, Affections, c.22, 43.

[143] John Gilbert entered the Blues as a lieut., 17 June 1712; capt.-lieut., 20 Jan. 1731; capt., 20 April 1732. He remained with the regiment until it returned to England in 1746, but appears to have left soon thereafter. WO 64/10, f. 8; *Army List of 1740*, p. 6.

[144] Horace, Satires, 2.7.102–3.

[145] Horace, Epistles, 1.20.10.

[146] Ibid., 9.13.

upon breaking open he recovered. Aprl. 20th Sr James Chamberlayne had a slight gout in wrists & anckles & has been often laid up six weeks at home; here was only confined a few days & advised the following medicine by way of prevention:

[*margin:* a preservative medecine.] {**Take 1 oz. of powdered gum guaiacum and 4 oz. of oily salt of vitriol; mix, and extract a tincture over 4 days, shaking frequently, then let the clear liquid be poured out and kept for use, 60 drops to be taken twice a day on sugar.**}

This was sometimes made in rum for the same purpose, is said to be originally from Dr. Boerhaave.[147] both he & Captn. Gilbert say it does them good by keeping the *body* open. the parts remained weake some time ({**"also weakens the feet and makes them feeble."**})[148] Some apply raw flesh to the affected part, which eases the pain, but acting as a repellant is often attended with bad consequence[x]. vid: Car: Piso obs: med: pag: 398.[149]

160.

[x]vid: Biograph: Britannic: Art: Betterton. vol.2d. p.779.[150]

161. [*continuing from p. 159*]

Coll: Beake had it in the right foot about the heel & anckle, June 5th 1743. has had it often & violently; thinks it's occasioned from drinking the small Rhenish & Moselle wines; is subject to shaking of the hand which is worse since he came to this country. this held him only a few days & was slight; its his custom to purge with Daffies Elixr. & takes Gum: Guajac & Sal: V. Oleos:

({**"So it's right we old fellows should gratify other old fellows."**} Ter: heau Act:3. Scen:1. V:10.[151])

about the same time Sr James had a slight touch in the right wrist, says rubbing the part with common treacle assuages the pain but never tryed

---

[147] It is possible that Boerhaave did indeed provide this formula, though it does not appear in his *Aphorisms* or in his *Materia Medica; or, a Series of Prescriptions* (London: W. Innis [etc.], 1741).

[148] Provenance unknown.

[149] Le Pois, *Selectiorum observationum*, p. 398 (sect. v, cap. i ["Of Arthritis"]). Le Pois asserts that when venesection is applied in the body part opposite the pain, it causes a revulsion, which reduces pain and increases blood flow. In Le Pois' experience, the relief of pain is most certain when the amount of blood taken is large.

[150] Reference is to the actor and dramatist Thomas Betterton, who according to Buchanan's source died from a revulsion, after he applied medicines to his feet in an effort to relieve swelling caused by gout: *Biographia Britannica: or, The Lives of the Most Eminent Persons Who have Flourished in Great Britain and Ireland, from the Earliest Ages, down to the Present Times* (London: W. Innys [etc.], 1748), II, 779.

[151] Terence, Self-tormentor 3.419.

it. there's but one Soldier in the Regmt troubled with this disease, viz: Campbell of Captn. Loyd's troop, an Argyleshire man & is hereditary.

{"Healing art knows not how to remove crippling gout, it helps not the fearful dropsy."}

Ov: de Ponto lib:1 V.255.[152]

[*margin:* many Gouty Officers but few soldiers] there's not a Regmt in the Service without two or three Gouty Officers but it's rare to see a gouty Soldier & they seldom or never breed it. vid: Buch: Eleg: ad Ptolemaeum Luxeum Tastaeum &c:[153] Sr James had it in his feet febry. 1746 & held him some weeks, thought

162. [*facing p. 161; blank*]

163. [*continuing from p. 161*]
it proceeded from lying cold the night we embarked for England, his feet being wet.

[*margin:* the Gout not occasioned from drinking French wines.] When at home our Gouty Officers avoid drinking French wines, for fear of giving them the Gout. but in Flanders it's the only wine they drink, particularly Burgundy, Hermitage & acknowledge they never were so healthy. & in our Dutch cantoonment French claret was drunk dayly & that freely, yet I don't remember many Gouty complaints.

[*margin:* evacuations necessary in the Gout.] Gouts from a Surfeit or hard living in a Sanguine constitution require evacuations: Cpt. Loyd was laid up some days at Coventry & confined to his bed or chair, his anckles useless & wrists so weake that he could not hold a small book.[154] was briskly purged with Pil: coc: min. & Cal: on the purging day he could walk with pleasure & lift a chair, but nixt day was weake, but recovered always with purging. & this was my constant practice with Sir John Bennet,[155] being of a Sanguine constitution & Subject to fevers. have

---

152 Ovid, Ex Ponto, 1.3.24–5.

153 Buchanan's fourth elegy, "Ad Ptolemaeum Luxium Tastaeum, & Jacobum Tevium cum articulari morbo laboraret" ("To Ptolemaeus Luxius Tastaeus and Jacobus Tevius, while he was ill with a disease of the joints"), was written in 1544, during an extended illness that he suffered while in Paris; in it, he describes at length the symptoms of his disease, including weakness and pain. Translation and discussion in David Henry Sabrio, "George Buchanan's *Elegies* and *Silvae* translated, with Introduction and Commentary" (unpub. Ph.D. diss., Univ. of South Carolina, 1980), pp. 66–73.

154 John Loyde or Lloyd was commissioned a cornet in the Blues 3 April 1718; a lieut., 12 Dec. 1728; a capt.-lieut., 25 April 1741; and a capt., 27 May 1742. He left the regiment in late 1753. RADCP, box 3/47; WO 27/1, 2, 3, 4, returns for Blues; *AL 1740*, p. 6.

155 Sir John Bennett, bart., entered the Blues as a cornet, 5 Feb. 1706; lieut., 24 Nov. 1715; capt.-lieut., 20 April 1732; capt., 29 Jan. 1734. He sold his commission 27 May 1742 and died at Fifes 28 April 1752. WO 64/10, f. 7; *LM*, XXI (1752), 239.

blooded, clystered &c. & always succeeded. A Gentleman having the Gout in his great toe, & vexed with pain, scarified it with his penknife, blooded a small quantity to his present relief.

{**"Inasmuch as this [i.e. corruption of blood by bile and phlegm]** [*continues on p. 165*]

164. [*facing p. 163; blank*]

165. [*continuing from p. 163*]
takes place in vessels that are the finest and by nature most critical in the body, as well as in sinews and bones that are many and dense, the condition is most persistent and intractable."} Hip: de Affect.[156]

{**"For goutish pain, apply to the swelling ground nitre mixed with water into a cataplasm, and do not wash it off for three days, but when you wash it, put on crude red nitre with a little honey. Use this, as it were, always."**} Ib: de mor. mulier: lib:1.[157]

[*margin:* Consumptions.] Par: 22. Consumptive people are more healthie here than at home; live much on vegetables, all garden herbs being in great abundance & good of their kind, abstaine from malt liquor: drinking wine & water.

[*margin:* Method of Cure.] are treated with pectorals, warm milk & Cons: rosar:

{**"Let the patient also drink raw cow's milk, to which one-third part of honeyed water has been added, for 45 days, and mix marjoram with it as well .... It is a serious disease, and few escape it."**} Hip: de intern: affect:[158]

Night sweats keep the patient very weake. The Bark the best remedy taken with a slight bitter wine. Some men swallow two or three Young frogs or snails on a morning without any sickness at Stomach or any other effects. Cpt. Forbes's[159] Servant has swallowed Dozens.

[*margin:* Hospital practice.] in the Hospital frequent bleedings were tryed in small

166. [*facing p. 165; blank*]

167. [*continuing from p. 165*]

---

156 Hippocrates, Affections, c.31.

157 Hippocrates, Diseases of Women, 1.98.

158 Hippocrates, Internal Affections, c.10.

159 Hugh Forbes was born c.1701 and gained a commission as cornet (at a comparatively advanced age) 18 July 1737; lieut.; 17 Feb.1741; capt., 23 July 1745; major, 17 Dec. 1756; sold his commission and retired, 29 Dec. 1758. WO 27/4, 5; WO 64/10, f. 7; *AL 1758*, p. 17.

quantities viz: from oz. iv. to oz. vi. prescribing Saponaceous medecines in large quantities, making Seatons in each side of the breast about 2. inches below the nipple: these Seatons discharge largely & I have seen some recover to admiration, were formerly walking Skeletons now fat & plump & free from Cough. if the cough proves at any time unease, bleeding is immediately repeated. Dr. Pringle took to this method from observing the lungs of consumptives to be wasted or useless from tubercles &c: & of consequence not sufficient to *ventilate the blood.* therefor proposed lessening, the mass at different times, that the lungs might be able to do their duty on the remaining part. Some were blooded nineteen times in Six weeks. I suspected these Seatons would produce carious ribs, which never happened, for they always worked outwards towards the skine.

[*margin:* Consumptives & phthisickey people are better in field than in Garrison.] Consumptive & pthisicky people are always better in field, than in Garrison, providing their Duty be moderate, a plain proof of the ben*e*fite of horse exercise so much recommended by Sydenhame. three recovered in Campn 1745 from milk dyet and pil: pectoral: nostr. with gentle rieding. one was attended with Spitting of blood & recovered by frequent bleedings in small

168. [*facing p. 167; blank*]

169. [*continuing from p. 167*]
quantities. (vid: Cornaro de la Sante des Princes. p.96[160]).

> {**"This man should be given hellebore and a decoction of lentils and as much food as possible, but should abstain from pungent flesh, beef, pork, and mutton; he should do a few exercises and take walks, and afterwards should vomit; he should refrain from sex."**} Hipp: de morb: lib.2.[161]

Qr. Mr. Wilcox[162] is Riding-Master to the Regmt, naturally fat & corpulent, during the winter grows fat & purcy, big bellyed, becomes indolent for want of exercise. when our recruite horses are brought over nixt Spring, he has then hard exercise in breaking Young horses and teaching Young men to ride, is dayly a horseback, soon looses his big

---

160 Bernardino Ramazzini, *L'art de conservar la santé des princes* (Leiden, 1724) [note: The volume that provides this translation into French of Ramazzini's *De principum valetudine tuenda* also includes *Les avantages de la vie sobre*, by Luigi Cornaro; Buchanan may have been confused about the authorship of *La santé de princes*].

161 Hippocrates, Diseases, II, c.49.

162 William Wilcox was commissioned a cornet in the Blues, and a quartermaster and riding master, 25 April 1741. He remained with the regiment at least until 1755. His difficulty with ulcerated legs is noted below, *ms.p. 203.* RADCP, Box 3/47; *AL 1754*, p. 61.

belly, grows more active every day, & as he expresses it, is fit to jump over the moon & a Stomach to eat a piece of a dead horse. & some of our men seem to be in the last stage of this distemper & uncapable of Garrison Duty, looking more fit for an hospital than a camp, yet recover wonderfully when in the field.

[*margin:* Venereale Desease.] Par: 23. It is a common notion that Venereal disorders are more malignant here than at home, but I have not had sufficient observation to form any just judgement. Some Buboes from England were more virulent than one could well imagine, having been twice fluxed in the hospital, fumigated with

170. Venereal cases were more malignant in Brussells than at Ghent, commonly appearing at first with shankers, excoriations, Buboes, parts swelled, all complaints virulent. Mercurial Vomits were used more freely, to some I have given dr.fs. & never any bad complaint. they were more mild in Germany, being only Simple Gonorheas.

171. [*continuing from p. 169*]

Cinnabar &c: yet far from being well tho Patient seems to be in a good State of health. it's a difficult task to cure the private men of claps: when the pain<full> symptoms abate, they neglect taking medecines, let the running continue till it turns to a Gleet, then say they were not well cured.

[*margin:* Officers more easely cured than the men.] Officers are more easely cured & that with the very same medecines being more carefull of health & keeping a proper Regimen.

[*margin:* Gonorhea.] The Gonorhea appears in the Space of a week after infection & may <be> caught by touching the parts only without coition as was the case of No. 3. and No. 5. says he got it going to the same necessarie house where two of his clapped Comrades frequented[a].

[*margin:* Method of Cure.] I commonly begin with calomel purges & continue till the running grow thick & white. the common purge is Jalap & Sal: Prunella & for heat of urine {**Sal prunella and white sugar, in the same quantities, as much as is required.**} taken frequently in a Glass warm water or whey, marsh mallow tea with Gum Arabic: Lintseed tea with Sal: Prunel: &c: I reckon the desease about half cured when the above complaints cease, & then order pil: resinos: nostr. or an Electuary with G. Guajac: Rhab. with tereb. Venet. &c: which operate by wine & keep the body open; towards the latter

172. [a]No.1. caught it tho he had a natural Phimosis, & the orifice so very small, that it was only sufficient to pass the urine. No.2 from the woman's handling the part only, thinks she rubbed some matter brought from her own Body.

{**"Wherefore, that you may have no reason to repent, cease to court matrons, for thence one may derive pain and misery, rather than reap enjoyment in the reality. Though this may not be your opinion, Cerinthus, yet not softer or finer are a woman's limbs amidst snowy pearls and green emeralds – nay, often the advantage is with the strumpet."**}

Hor: Sat:2. lib:1. V:77.[163]

{**"In a matron one can only see her face, for unless she be a Catia, her long robe conceals all else."**}

Ib. et vid. Ep.17. lib.1. V:55.[164]

173. [*continuing from p. 171*]
end, advise the cold bath or washing with cold water.

[*margin:* never use injections.] seldom or never use injections, & never saw one of our men have a Caruncle:

[*margin:* the men are irregular as to Regimen, & love to be heartely worked.] are well in Six or Seven weeks tho very irregular as to Regimen, their breakfast is water gruell, with which they work on their physick which procures a good appetite for dinner & eat freely of mess food with their Comrades & rarely abstaine from drinking. they love to be heartely worked & Jalap answers this purpose working briskly & seldom attended with grieps, there's a vulgar & unjust prejudice against it from being cheap & so much in practice. Manna & Salts is the common method with officers, giving calomel pill overnight; repeated every other day, & with this have only made a cure in three weeks time; but the men don't think this strong enough.

[*margin:* Cordee] The Cordee is one of the most troublesome complaints,

[*margin:* method of cure.] rubbing with Ungt. merial [*sic*] is of use, or dissolved {**In eggyolk with barley water.**} & injected. I often prescribe thus. {**Take 4 gr. turbith mineral and 6 gr. each of calomel and camphor and as much lenitive electuary as is necessary to make a bolus.**}[.] it's purgative, seldom emetick; & if often repeated makes a sore mouth. Mercuric vomits are often given for this purpose. I often use them in venerale cases & never saw anything dangerous attending them as

174. [*facing p. 173; blank*]

---

[163] Horace, Satires, 1.2.77–82.

[164] Ibid., 1.2.94–5; *Horace* (trans. Fairclough), p. 27. Epistles 17.1.55–8 translates, "[a complaining travel companion] recalls the familiar tricks of a mistress who oft bewails a pretty chain, oft a stolen anklet, so that by and by her real losses and griefs win no belief"; *Horace* (trans. Fairclough), p. 365.

175. [*continuing from p. 173*]
is commonly reported. I once knew a violent Cordee relieved by accidental bleeding from the part & have always thought bleeding with a Leech would be of Service, but none incline to try. Sometime after the running stops & the patient quite well, there remains pain & heat round the os pubis greatly alarming the patient, though never of any bad consequence & easely removed by any lenient purge.

[*margin:* Phimosis.] The Phimosis is often troublesome both to Patient & Surgn.

[*margin:* Method of Cure.] fomentations are necessary. warm milk, rubbing with ungt. mercurial or injection as above. our men often use warm small beer & butter & some fat broth, & always bread & milk poultice. Peerage, of Col. Beakes's had it to a great degree & would not suffer anything to be done, being a Farrier only rubbed with Ungt. Dealth. & continued so two years, laughing that he now got a natural scabbard, & swearing he would never draw his sword. was lately discharged. we had many in Garrison 1744 & some required the operation.

[*margin:* Paraphimosis.] Paraphimosis more dangerous than the above, sometimes threatning a mortification, the Glans swelling to a great size, pustules rise & containe a sharp water, excoriating &c[;] the above method usefull, yet the operation cannot be avoided in some cases. or slight incisions where the stricture is strongest

176. [*facing p. 175; blank*]

177. [*continuing from p. 175*]
rubbing the Glans with brandy & oyle; some use cold water & vinegar. this often happens after recovering a Phimosis, being fond of pulling the prepuce back before it is sufficiently relaxed, catches the Glans suddenly, & sometimes so tight that the urine cannot pass.

[*margin:* Swelled testicles.] Swelled testicles are frequent, & said to be occasioned from astringent medecines & the Surgeon always blamed; but are rather from catching cold, riding, intemperate drinking & private debauches, & are very obstinate in old venereal constitutions as was with Barbier of Sir James's, continued six weeks notwithstanding a gentle *Sale.* bleeding &c. as above are necessary & turpeth vomits of great use. when the swelling decreases the part should be keep'd warm, wearing a truss of flannel &c. otherwise it returns on the least Cold. small hard knotty lumps adhering to the testicle remain some time, & the Strings are often hard & as it were twisted, but of no dangerous consequence. warm milk & honey is a favorite fomentation with some, greatly asswages pain.

[*margin:* Shankers.] Shankers often appear without any other Symptoms, are taken off with Scissars, cut down with Causticks, Vitriol:

Rom: or Lint. ad ulcera venerea nostr. dissolving them insensibly without pain & have been often surprized at its good success.

178. [*facing p. 177; blank*]

179. [*continuing from p. 177*]
I have seen the whole Glans covered like a Cluster of Grapes & cured without pain. great care should be taken in order to keep the neighbouring parts clean for the matter breeds others or makes large excoriations.

{**"And fires neglected are wont to gather strength."**}
Hor: Ep.18. lib:1. V:85.[165]

Women often neglect them till they become filthy ulcers.

{**"Fools, through false shame, hide the unhealed sore."**}
Ep.16. lib.i. V:24.[166]

internale medecines as above are usefull, but our troopers are careless & if the ulcer be healed, they never think of taking physick, but quite otherwise with Officers. Paterson of the King's had many ulcers & was a careless dirty fellow, not keeping them clean[;] was prisoner in the hole three days & fed on bread & water only. on coming out the parts were quite clean tho never dressed.

[*margin:* Buboes.] Buboes often appear without any preceeding Symptom; sometimes sooner or later. our fellows are such dablers that there's nothing certain to be learned from them.

[*margin:* Method of Cure.] so soon as they appear I apply Empl: Diachyl: c: Gum:, allowing the fellow to live as usuale & take his Pot of Beer. their custom is to drink Gin but that makes them drunk & does not answer the intention. some ripen of themselves without any application. some are kindly & do well without much trouble. those of a healthy strong constitution ripen

180. [*facing p. 179; blank*]

181. [*continuing from p. 179*]
best & such as live well. Some fellows are drunkish every night & have told me it cost them a Ducate to nurse their pig & make it ready for the knife. when ripe I open with the Lancet, cutting off the edges: dress with dry Lint, covering with digestive. if the edges grow hard and callous, rub with Ungt. mercurial; if proud flesh touch with Caustic or Vitriol: Rom: if foul at bottom, sprinkle praecipt. rubr. or Ungt. Aegyptiac; when opened by Caustic, the business is done at once, seldom proud flesh or callous edges, but the men have not the patience for Caust: some are faint

[165] Horace, Epistles, 1.18.85.

[166] Ibid., 1.16.24.

& sicke as from bleeding. others never mind it, making no complaint, riding dayly, only lying by a day or two when near ripe, and some are so large that they cannot walke upright, but crawl on their hands & feet. Some complaine of so much pain as not suffer You to touch it. are even afraid if You look at it, and people of this constitution are always a long time a curing. Paterson of the King's in naturally of a sulkie temper and must have repeated orders from his Corporale before he does his duty. The constitution of his body is much the same with respect to physick requiring almost double Doses to operate, is now fluxing & has double the quantity of Mercury that others have. I seldom attempt to disperse them.

182. [*facing p. 181; blank*]

183. [*continuing from p. 181*]

[*margin:* not always confined to the Groine.] they may happen in other parts of the body as well as in the Groine & Crosfield of Coll. Beake's had one on the os pubis, Attree of Major Jenkinson's in the arm pit, & in another on the fore part of the neck.

[*margin:* are easier cured than claps.] I would rather undertake the cure of Bubo than that of a Clap. so long as they require dressing the men attend dayly for fear of being poxed, & never pretend to cure themselves; but their private receipts for claps are infinite. when the cure is compleated they don't mind physick or any regimen, but return to the old way, & if poxed thereafter blame their Surgeon. Some do not heal kindly, continue ouzing from a small orifice; & some have small sinuses of this kind, threatning to be fistulous. Should be laid open with Lancet or Caustic: applyed, if compress & bandage faile.

[*margin:* not to be opened till ripe.] I have imagined Buboes might be opened by Caustic befor they were quite ripe, & that the discharge after the Eschar cast off would be sufficient, & by this method shorten the cure, not waiting for Suppuration; but then the Gland remains undestroyed, having never suppurated; is hard, proves tedeous work to the Surgn & great pain to the patient; escarotick powders must be applied, viz: <pulv.> Angelic: round the root of the Gland, pressing the

184. [*facing p. 183; blank*]

185. [*continuing from p. 183*]

dressings tight towards the bottom, in order to root it out, & some cut it out as soon as they can get at it. others waste with Caustic, continuing a course of internal mercurials. Rylie of the King's Troop had one on our March to Germany & promising to ripen, encreasing dayly; at Maestrict we received ammonition bread, & proved purgative at first, being mixed with a large quantity of Rye; he was violently purged and the Bubo disappeared. his dyet was Spare, sweating much from the heat of weather & exercise, & never had other complaint.

[*margin:* Venereal Eruptions.] Venereal eruptions on the Skin are common amongst us, and I have often been afraid to attempt a cure without salivating from the difficulty represented by Practical Authors, but our men have neither time nor Patience for this method. & I have often thought of trying some uncommon mercurial preparation for this purpose.

[*margin:* Method of Cure.] the best I know are our pil: Mercurial: nostr. taking two morning & evening, desisting if the mouth or Gums grow sore, & begin again when that goes off, been often surprized at their good success. two or three Dozen has done wonders & that without any visible operation; & some have taken three Dozen without the least soreness of mouth. mercurial Oynt. should be used externally with prudence. I have tryed several mercurial

186. [*facing p. 185; blank*]

187. [*continuing from p. 185*]
preparations, but never found any more effectual than the above. I deflagrated Mercur: precipt: rubr. dr.ii with Brandy three times, finely prepared in a marble mortar & formed into pills ad: gr.i aut ii. are purgative, making a slight sickness at Stomach, taking one morning & evening & sometimes raise a slight spitting; one man took twenty two in ten days, without any remarkable operation; had many venereal Blotches, shankers, aching pains in the bones & did well; was surprised to see so great an alteration from so small a Pill. Fishar of Col. Beake's his skin was covered over & of long standing, dry Scales &c.

> **{"The dark colour and the black spots on her breast in front were signs that her heart is not without stain of unfaithfulness."}**
>
> Ov. Amor: lib:ii. eleg.:c. V:43.[167]

& C.F:[168] took them in our Dutch cantoonment during the hard frost, with the same good effect. Turpeth. mineral: prepared in the same manner answered the same purpose. our men only found fault with them as being so small and having no violent operation, imagining medecines can have no good effect unless they be rough in their operation. Small doses Calomel has the same effect. continued some time and raising a slight Salivation, called a <u>walking Sale</u>. the men walk abroad dayly taking care to keep the feet dry, wearing two

167 Ovid, Amores, 3.5.43–4.

168 Possibly Captain Forbes (cf. n. 159).

188. [*facing p. 187; blank*]

189. [*continuing from p. 187*]
shirts or flannel westcoat, their cloake &c., walking in the Sun in order to sweat, all sweat largely in the night from drinking something warm at bedtime &c. their chief dyet is water gruelle with bread in which they boyle Young nettle tops. Elder buds &c: making Spring pottage as in England, with which they wash the mouth frequently. Some require three or four Scruples befor the mouth grow sore, others flux sufficiently with half the quantity, & some are always purged, & all attended with the same good effect. which is to be continued till all complaints cease; the skin should be washed dayly with a Sponge & soapie water, well rub'd. warm bathing would be of great service. abstaining from Salt or fat meats. Murrel of Sr James took thirty three pills aa. gr.v: fluxed gently, his mouth never sore, and purged dayly. Harding of Captn. Gilbert's took upwards of fourty in March & Aprl. many others were treated in this manner & all succeeded. & I have observed fewer relapses after this slow method than from higher Salivations. & tho in cold rooms there has not been the least bad consequence, but irregular fellows are not to be trusted in this manner. when the head is scabbed they rub the part too freely with Ungt. Mercurial, from seeing its good affects on other parts & sometimes

190. [*facing p. 189; blank*]

191. [*continuing from p. 189*]
throw themselves into a high salivation, & befor it can be checked the hair is obliged to be taken off, to the great grief of the Trooper. I have also used mer praecipt. pr. Se with the same success.

[*margin:* Nocturnale pains.] Nocturnal Pains are seldom alone, something Venereal appearing to the Eye; tho Some Soldiers magnify complaints of this kind even after a regular Salivation in hopes of being discharged, but have been frequently detected as impostors. are to <be> treated in the above manner, tho Salivation is their last recourse, which is always in the Hospital & chiefly by unction[a].

[*margin:* Nodes & Exostoses.] Nodes & Exosdoses render the Soldier unfit for Duty, cannot <bear> a boot &c: & as he is likely to be so for a long time, is more proper for the Hospital than his quarters. the common practice is to apply caustic to the part. a large Eschar is cast off, the bone rasped & chiselled in order to take off all that is affected, & unless You go to the bottom You are dayly plagued with filthy Spungie excrescences. dress with pledgits in Mastich: &c. covering with digestives. these caustics require much time & give great pain & after all there's much work for the knife. I would therefor prefer the incision at first. Nodes & exostoses remaine after Salivation, & should be crushed in the bud.

192. [a][*margin:* method of fluxing in the hospital.] the method of fluxing in our hospital is first to bleed, purge & bath. The Pa<tients> are dressed in flannel resembling the dress of a Capuchine; confined to a warm room, & always raised by unction viz: one 3d. Argt. viv: ad Axung: Porcin: rubbing dr.i. on legs & thighs h.S: nixt night the same quantity on the arms, then the lower extremities, & repeated every night till the Spitting begin, which is commonly after the 3d. or 4th rubbing, amounting to three pots in 24 hours. each pot containing about a pint English. Some require a turpeth vomite to raise it & is afterwards keeped up by small doses Calomel, rubbing the part afected dayly with Ungt. Mercurial & continuing till the complaints are quite gone. some times it goes off by urine and Sweat, & attended by the same good effect as Spitting. if grieps or purging are troublesome Decoct. Diascord. & Op. are used, Decoct. Alb. or Gum: Arab: theire ordinary drink. their chief food Ryce Gruell, light bread pudding & their common drink barley water, water Gruell &c. when the Salivation is finished, they are put on a course of the wood Decoction, taking Gum. Guajac. and Argt. viv: in pills, &seldom faile of a cure. Some years ago this was looked on as the utmost danger & of the greatest consequence & called the Grand Cure, always under the care of Physicians of the greatest experience, now mostly under the Surgeones or their Mates & seldom attended with bad consequence. yet one of our men died at Brussells, being jaw-locked.

193. [*continuing from p. 191*]

old Venereals & much emaciated have recovered & able to do Duty from this method being keep'd strickly to a long course of Mercurials & wood-Drinks. others are walking Skeletons for life[a].

> **{"His passion made him lean: his legs between the joints are long, his long neck is still long, his head is far from his body."}**
> Ov: met: lib:12. V:794.[169]

Heskin's Coll. Beake's, had a large excrescence on the upper lip which almost obstructed his nostrills, & many large dry scabs cast off. being an old Venereal I treated with mercurials in small Doses rubbing the part with this Oynt. {Take 2 dr. mercurial ointment and mix with ½ scr. corrosive sublimate.} & dissolved dayly.

[*margin:* Imaginary Venereals.] We have many imaginary Venereals, & when one of a Troop is fluxed for venereale complaints, if any of his old Companions have the least aching pain in their bones from catching cold or scabs on their skin from itch or scurvy, presently

[169] Ovid, Metamorphoses, 11.793–4.

reflecting on their past life, conclude themselves poxed & are not satisfied without fluxing. Marriote of the Major's when confined from a broken leg a lying in the ward nixt the Salivating, & many Venereal Patients lying in the same roome, & often relating their Cases; imagined he was poxed & could not be satisfyed without a Salivation, which he had, tho there was no appearance of any Venereal taint: & some are so intent on fluxing that they are fluxed from imagination

194.

[a] {**"Solomon tells the young men to avoid consorting with strange women, 'Lest thou mourn at the last, when thy flesh and thy body are consumed.'"**} Prov: C.5. V:xi.[170]

{**"Excessive sex swiftly ages a woman and causes her to become greatly disfigured and ugly."**} Perer: in Genes: C: 20, Disput. i.[171]

{**"To see all this is salvation to a young man."**}

Ter. Eun: Act:5. S:4. V.184.[172]

{**"For an intemperate and indulgent youth delivers to old age a body all worn out."**}

Tull: de Senect.[173]

195. [*following on p. 193*]
only. as was the case of a Soldier in the first Regimt of Guards Decr. 1743. imagining himself poxed & insisting on a Salivation. upon examination at the Hospital nothing appeared Venereal. Complaints were Scorbutick and Rheumatick. but he would be fluxed & in order to please him was put into the fluxing dress, viz: flannel shirt & Drawers &c. orderd. to keep very warm & taste nothing that was cold. as there was no bed for him in the Fluxing Ward, was told he was to be put under a Mercuriale Course & have a walking Sale in a proper ward with all necessary care, begging him to be very cautious as to eating & drinking &c:

[*margin:* Imaginary flux.] Crude antimony was given in form of an Elect: directed the mercurial Elect: &c: which he took with great care and pleasure, expecting a fine cure; in a few days he began to spit, imagined his teeth loose & mouth sore, & fluxed a good pint a day & extreamely happy at the thoughts of doing so well. & this Salivation was lowered by degrees by lessing the Dose &c: & never was near the Salivating Ward. vid: Tulp: Ob: p. 35,93.[174] & Ov: rem: Amor. V.525.

---

170 Proverbs 5:11.

171 Benito Pereira [Benedictus Pererius], *Commentarium et disputationum in Genesim* (Coloniae Aggripinae, 1601), cap. xx, disp. i (t. 3 [vol. II], 891)(V, 525).

172 Terence, Eunuchus, 5.940.

173 Cicero, de Senectute, 9.29.

174 Tulp, *Observationes medicae*, I, pp. 35, 93.

{**"For since natures vary, I will vary my arts; the disease has a thousand forms, I have a thousand remedies."**}[a].[175]

Montaigne's Essays chap: XX on the force of Imagination.[176] Turner's Siphyllis.[177]

Burford of Majr: Jenkinson's taking pil: pect: nostr. for a Cough, was perswaded by his Comrades they were Mercurials. nixt *day* began to Spit largely, when increased to a great degree, guessed at two pints a day, neither

196.

[*margin:* triffling cases not to be sent to the hospital.] [a]Surgeons should not send triffling cases to an hospital: those who go for slight Surgery cases are in great danger of catching some distemper of the house viz. fever, small pox &c. Harris of Cpt. Shipman's having dislocated his collar bone attended with great contusion was sent to Tournay hospital; got a slowe fever with great variety of complaints, took a dislike to the house from seeing so many disagreeable objects, continued in a lingring way some months, was at last brought to his Barracks at Brussels, tho we had a good Hospital there, would not be perswaded to go to it, but chose to die in his qtrs always thinking of what he had seen in the hospital. Some are naturally lazy & indolent & are much more so after being some time in the hospital. Some pretend to be sick or Lame & uncapable of Duty but can do some work in the hospital when employed as servants, & have good wages. these are not easely detected, tho sometimes discovered by making them drunk, & carefully observing their motions. a Stiff Knee is a common complaint, but upon being fudled, can dance, jump, & cut capars.

({**"What a miracle cannot the wine-cup work."**} Hor: Ep.5. lib:i.[178])

Some suffer the part to be blistered, Seatons cut &c: but have recovered upon hearing the Surgeons whisper that a red hot iron must be applied for nine mornings in order to remove that humor from the bone. a foot

---

175 Ovid, Cure for Love, v.525–6.

176 Although Buchanan refers to the essay (bk. I, ch. 20) in general, he may have had in mind comments like the following: "We sweat, we shake, we grow pale, and we blush at the motions of our imaginations; and wallowing in our beds we feel our bodies agitated and turmoiled at their apprehensions, yea in such manner, as sometimes we are ready to yeeld up the spirit." Michel de Montaigne, *The Essays of Montaigne*, trans. John Florio, introd. J. I. M. Stewart (New York: The Modern Library, n.d.), p. 64.

177 Daniel Turner, *Syphilis: A Practical Dissertation on the Venereal Disease*, 4th ed., rev. (London: J. Walthoe [etc.], 1732). On pp. 121–37, Turner discusses the case histories of four men who consulted him because they were convinced that they were suffering from venereal disease.

178 Horace, Epistles, 1.5.16.

Guard, by trade a taylor & Perruque maker was in the hospital for a fistula in Ano, had good business in his own trade, & was better pleased to continue there than go to the field; but the fistula being almost well, was told he must think of joining his *Regmt.* but he contrived a method to keep the fistula always open by introducing a pea after the Surgeones dressing & taking it out nixt morning. but being drunk overnight, & dressed sooner nixt morning than he expected, was discovered & turned out. vid. Roderic. a Castro Medic: Politic: lib:4. C:9. Qua ratione Morbum Simulantes deprehendi queant.[179]

197. [*continues from p. 195*]:
mouth nor Gums sore, abstaining from the pills, salivation abated, was faint & weake as from violent purging. When the men have been often in for it, they are more cautious in their intrigues.

{**"For the wolf is wary and dreads the pit, the hawk the suspected snare, the pike the covered hook."**}

Hor: Ep.16. lib:i. V:50.[180]

{**"If the crow could feed in quiet, he would have more meat, and much less wrangling and envy."**}

Ib: Ep:17. lib:i V:50.[181]

[*margin:* Scurvy.] Par: 24th. Scorbuticke complaints are not so frequent as one would expect, as they are said to be predominant in every English constitution. but rare amongst our Troopers.

[*margin:* Method of Cure] at first I use mercurial purgatives, rubbing the Spots with Ungt. Mercur: putting them under a course of Aethiop: Mineral. Cornet Newton[182] is of a Scorbutick habite many red Spots at the bending of the arms & cannot abstaine from scratching. took Succ: Antiscorbutic: cum chalyb: was very regular in Dyet, eating Spring Sallads, watercresses &c. abstaining from high Sauces, rubbing the parts {**Take 1 oz. pomatum and 1 dr. white precipitate of mercury.**}. recovered dayly, drinking whey afterwards every morning for some weeks. Cpt. Marchame had it to the most violent degree I ever

---

179 Rodrigo de Castro [Rodericus a Castro], *Medicus-politicus: sive, De officiis medico-politicis tractatus, quatuor distinctus libris: in quibus non solum bonorum medicorum mores ac virtutes exprimuntur, malorum vero fraudes & imposturae deteguntur, verum etiam pleraque, alia circa novum hoc argumentum utilia atque iucunda exactissime proponuntur* (Hamburg: Bibliopolio Frobeniano, 1614), IV, cap. ix (pp. 251–4). In this chapter, the author discusses cases of feigned illness, madness—he notes Ulysses' attempt at deception—and injuries, and advises how frauds can be detected.

180 Horace, Epistles, 1.16.50–1.

181 Ibid., 1.17.50–1.

182 Charles Newton (b. c.1714) was commissioned a cornet in the Blues on 18 Sept. 1741; lieut., May 1745; capt.-lieut., Aug. 1753; capt., 22 Dec. 1753; sold out 14 June 1756. RADCP, Box 3/47; WO 27/4, return for Blues; *AL 1756*, p. 14.

saw, especially his thighs & forearms being covered with large dry hard blotches, itchy & burning hot, scaly skin like parchment, & crackled as I cut with my Lancet when

198. [*facing p. 197; blank*]

199. [*continuing from p. 197*]
bleeding. urine high coloured with a thick red Sandy Sediment, hot & scalding, making water often & in small quantity, restless & tossing in bed, great oppression at breast, was purged and put on a whey & vegetable Dyet, drinking scorbutic juices. {**Take 4 parts of the leaves of nasturtium and mix with 2 parts of equal quantities of becabunga and horseradish and 2 oz. of newly picked wild radish; express the juice according to art; of which let him take 4 spoonfuls with 1 spoonful lemon juice, 10 gr. vitriol martis, and 2 oz. of a generous Rhenish wine; to be taken every morning on an empty stomach, and whey to be drunk freely 4 times a day.**} bathed the parts affected with fomentation of Scorbutick plants rubbing with Ungt. Citrin: lived much on Sparrow Grass, Spinage & extremely regular in Dyet. recovered dayly, & was thought a great cure, he had been Scorbutick fourteen years. after the juices he drunk Lymington well water in Warwickshire, a strong purgative water. the Decoction of Quicksilver is much esteemed by Some, & is thus made. {**Take 4 oz. of purified mercury and 4 lbs. of spring water; boil down by half.**} the quicksilver never loses weight nor changes colour & I have fluxed with it after being several times used for this purpose.

Some Gentlemen keep two or three pounds of it in their horse trough, & <the> water is reckoned good to kill

200. [*facing p. 199; blank*]

201. [*continuing from p. 199*]
and destroys worms. a Gentleman much afflicted with the Scurvy & having almost los'd the use of his limbs, taken many medecines and drunk mineral waters to no purpose; observing his farcy horses recover on being soyled with Fetches, imagined their juice would have the same affect on himself, & took it without any success, making him very sicke at Stomach. at last followed an old Woman's advise taking two Spoonfulls of juice of water Parsnips every morning in warm milke, & recovered dayly, continued well many Years. when Scorbuticke juices become desagreable to the Stomach, (for few can bear them a long time), I then Substitute Aq: Benedict &: pil: mercurial: nostr. [*notation:* The Scorbutick Whey of Lond: Dispensary 1747. is a good Medecine as dyet Drink.]

[*margin:* Ulcers on the Legs.] Par: 25th. Ulcers on the legs are difficult to cure especially if of long standing, the edges callous &c: & tho they appear to the eye a meer triefle yet they are always tedeous & sometimes never cured. a Surgeon gets no credite by them; the men will not keep a proper Regimen; You can hardly perswade them to take a Dose or two physick, the good effect of which is soon overballanced by the nixt debauch[a]. they are to be dayly washed with something warm, the callosity pared off, making small incisions round the

202.

[a]"**For the most part, purging the bowels agrees with ulcers, as well as wounds of the head, belly, and joints, where there is danger of gangrene, in such cases as require sutures, and in those where [ulcers] spread and creep .... Often, moreover, wash the ulcer with a sponge and then dry lint is to be frequently applied to it, then at length such medicine as is seen to be useful is to be applied, either with or without a bandage .... In circular ulcers, if somewhat hollow, you must scarify all along their edges, or to the extent of half the circle, according to the natural stature of the man."**} Hipp: de ulcerib: S.vi.[183]

203. [*continuing from p. 201*]:
circumference, in order to make them unite & grow together, sprinkling praecipt. in order to bring on a digestion & resemble a fresh wound, covering with Digestive. the callosity often returns, must be treated as at first, rubbing ungt. Mercurial: Constitutions are often pockie & pil: Mercurial: Nostr: are of great use, when almost well it's a difficult task to skin them over, & Ungt. Diapomphol: with a few grains Mercur: Dulc. is a good healer[a]]. When cured they often breake out from the least triffling hurt, & great care should be taken to preserve them from external injuries. the method is folding brown paper into many doubles and wearing it under the Stocking. some beat a lead bullet into a thin plate, others have a plate of tine lynned with soft leather to keep off the pressure of the boot &c. Ulcers of long continuance become natural issues. & being suddenly healed or dryed up produce bad symptoms viz: headachs, sickness at heart &c: & I have been obliged to make a fresh sore & waite a more favourable opportunity in order to cure them, as was the case of Hans of Cpt. Loyde's troop. amongst old women a poultice of Bay leaves boyled in milk is an infallible remedy for old ulcers; Qr. Mr. Wilcox tryed it, but not succeeding was cured as above. The men ride or walk dayly,

204.

---

[183] Hippocrates, Ulcers, c.2 and 3.

[a] {**"When you wish to bring the lips of the ulcer together, prepare the leaves of the *rosa canina* [dog rose] as you would the lentil or nasturtium (called *suridion* [in Greek]), and mix it with wine and powdered linseed. Also, macerate linseed, crude chaste tree, and Melian alum in vinegar."**} Hip: de ulcerib. S:vi.[184]

205. [*continuing from p. 203*]:
despising such small sores, & find fault with their Surgn for not curing them; these men when confined to the Hospital, are obliged to keep to their roome & lye on bed so many hours a day, are soon cured by this method[a].

[*margin:* Ulcers on the Sternum.] Ulcers of the Sternum & ribs are often attended with carious bones & seldom cured; are often the consequence of small abcesses in these parts.

[*margin:* & in urethra.] Venereal ulcers of the Urethra are difficult of cure. Derwen of Col. Beake's was Six weeks in the Hospital & under a mercurial course all that time, & not the better. on coming to his quarters used an injection of Lap: medicamentos: which dried the running some measure but did not cure it.

[*margin:* broken shins.] Par: 26. Broken-shins are very common amongst us, from kicks by the horses, falling throw Steps of the leather in going to the Hayloft, &c: the flesh often stripped from the bone & laid bare some inches, as was the case of Burry of Cpt. Gilbert's, his horse running against a post, the tibia was bare three inches, the fleshy part hanging down, being almost ready to drop off; Instances happen dayly both to Troopers & Ban-men.

[*margin:* Method of Cure.] I commonly dress with Bals: Universal: covering with digestive: having first replaced the tore flesh into its natural situation, if the neighbouring parts are much bruised, inflammed or painfull, foment & poultice. if the Surface of the bone be

206.

[a] {**"But to stand with an ulcer is not fitting, especially if that ulcer is situated in the leg; but neither, also, should one sit or walk. But quiet and rest are most beneficial."**} Hip de ulcerib: S.vi.[185]

vid Hoffmanni Op: Med: Tom.2. p443. de omnis generis Ulceribus tam benignis quam malignis praesertum Cancroris [186]

---

[184] Ibid., c.4.

[185] Ibid., c.1.

[186] "Regarding sores of all types, benign as well as malignant ones and especially cancerous ones": Hoffmann, *Opera omnia*, III, cap. vii, pp. 443–59. Hoffmann asserts that cancers arise from ulcers that have not been successfully treated. He defines different kinds of ulcers and recommends remedies.

207. [*continued from p. 205*]:

Smooth & no Splinter I suffer the flesh to cover as fast as possible, taking care not to wipe too hard for fear of destroying the growing flesh. in case of a rough surface or Splinters I keep open with Spunge tent, & waite their casting off; the edges grow hard and dry must be washed with something warm & greasie. the Stocking is a good & equal bandage[C], the leg to be raised up equal with the thigh, which is natural to the men as they sit or lye in their tents. must never ride or put on a boot. their Comrades think nothing of a broken shin, saying they have had as much at foot ball & cured it with a leafe of tobacco; grudge doing duty for their lame Comrade & often oblige him to do his Duty befor he is well. but in order to save him <I give> a certificate unfit for Duty a horse back directed to his Officer. Instances I could give many, but its needless. I have been often surprized at this Success, especially considering our manner of living & often walking abroad. Im [*sic*] persuaded many Surgeons by their overcare in wieping, probing, &c: often prolong the cure[a]. it's commonly said that a wound on an Englishman's leg is not easely cured, but I don't think them as bad as reported, tho many are Subject to swelled legs being full of humours

208.

[C] {**"But a linen cloth, rather loose, should first be applied to the swelling at the extremities; then it should be wound upwards, always stretched, avoiding constriction, but adapted so as to give the ulcer special support at the wound, but are less felt by the remaining parts.**} Hip: de fractis.[187] {"On the third day also [the dressings] should be loosened and tied again, but splints should not be used and even more than before, rest and refraining from food are necessary." Ib.[188]

[a] A horse's taile when nicked & sett, is commonly well in a fortnights time, tho the tendon be cut thro, & some part of it extracted; the first dressing is turpentine dissolved with the yolke of an egg & some tincture of Myrrh; this is continued the first three days, then untyed & suffered to fall off with the digestion, the wounds are then stroaked with a feather dipt in tinct: Myrrh: or Bals: Universal, & that only every 3d or 4th days.

209. [*continues from p. 207*]:

and like their greasie-heeled horses, purge them never so much will always swell.

[*margin:* Bruises.] Par: 27th[.] Bruises are common from the horse falling with his rider &c. & so violent that blood is sometimes squeezed

[187] Hippocrates, Fractures, c.27.

[188] Ibid.

from the toes, yet nothing broke nor dislocated. the part soon swells, turning black & blew; soon painfull & stiff.

[*margin:* Method of Cure.] the men rub immediately with Brandy & some use Spt. Vin: R: but is so dear here that is not much in fashion. I use Liniment: Vol: nostr: soaking brown paper, keeps the part moist & supple, assuaging pain, dispersing the swelling, though in some cases fomentations & poultices are necessary. & some use brandy & vinegar applyed very hot. others boyle Cow Dung in milk, slycing & dissolving soape & is an excellent poultice. Brandy & water make a good fomentation, & bread & milke the best poultice, tho very Simple yet keeps in vogue. Bleeding is usefull, especially if any bruise about the breast, head, &c. as in falls from horse backe, & so customary that on every slight fall or bruise the trooper thinks himself neglected if he is not blooded, many are fond of Irish Slate in Spruce beer, which I never used, but often prescribe Spermacet: & Sal V:C:C:, advising to live Sparingly on barley broths, drink whey &c. Bruises on the elbow are often troublesome forming into abcesses[;] in the head require large bleeding[;] are frequent in time

210. [*facing p. 209; blank*]

211. [*continuing from p. 209*]
of frost from falls on the Ice when learning to skeat or in the fields by falls with trusses of forrage. Black eyes are common from Blowes & bruises, the men ask cons: Ros[a?]r. & cure themselves, some apply roasted rotten apples; I often foment with warm milk in which elder or Chamomile flowers are boyled. with some a thin slice of raw veal is much esteemed to draw out the blackness, and much used amongst children. Brown paper soaked in oil and vinegar much in vogue with some[x]. <[x]others esteem fresh urine & Soap, & not without good reason.> Bruised toes are frequent from horses trampling on them, produce small abcesses & threatning the loss of the naile, Spirituous dressings are of service here, viz: linit: Myrrh: & al: or {**brandy or gin.**} Bruises on the Knee are very troublesome from the many membranes, tendons, Ligaments &c:

[*margin:* Sprains.] Par: 28th. Sprains are common as the above, viz: anckles, wrists, fingers &c: continue weake a long while.

[*margin:* Method of Cure.] the men are fond of Spt. Vin: & ol: tereb: Lint Vol: nostr. answer the purpose with proper bandage &c:

> {**"Where joints are dislocated or the nerves are twisted around them ... one should choose a bandage ... these bandages, compresses, etc. ... then extension, friction, adjustment, etc."**}
> Hip: de officina Medec:[189]

[189] Hippocrates, Physician, c.23.

recommending rest, the men have a great regard for Strengthening plaister, Searcloths & are never satisfyed without them[.] I have no esteem for them being perswaded these of the Shops are

212. [*facing p. 211; blank*]

213. [*continuing from p. 211*]
too hard a consistence for the heat of the body to dissolve any good quality from them. the French never use them. Brandy or Spt. of wine with Bandage & compress being their universal medicine. & it's customary with some of our Surgns to make good Strengthening plaisters out of the refuse of all others. but their chief use is to wear them six weeks or as long as they stick on, & during that time the part recovers strength. they are universally used by the common people of England & every private family had its own favourite Searcloth,[190] & are applyed to all aching pains, which are commonly called Sprains, never distinguishing twixt an inflammatory Stich or old Sprain, as happened to Gisline of Cpt. Maden's,[191] his Lieut. applyed his favorite Searcloth to a pleuretick Stich which he called a Sprain or Rench, & keeping it on some days, had almost cost the fellow his life for want of bleeding. cases of this kind I see dayly. as Stiches often proceed from violent exercise, running, leaping, jumping, throwing stones, the dealers in Searcloths name them Sprains or Renches, apply their never failing Searcloths, neglecting bleeding to the irreparable loss of the patient. the part continuing soft and numb, is to be put into warm Grains, or the paunch of a beast newly killed, keeping warm with flannel or fur, warm Soape Sudds, a good fomentation.

214. [*facing p. 213; blank*]

215. [*continuing from p. 213*]

> {**"Where the harm is, there especially one should press, therefore putting underneath soft wool underneath, suited to the affection. What is used should not excessively compress … but should be firm enough to prevent shaking [from coughs and sneezes], while not being too confining."**} Hip: de Officina Medeci[192]

[190] Cerecloths were cloths that had been dipped in a mixture of melted wax (hence, the name), oil of some sort, and often spices or other ingredients.

[191] James Madan (b. 1701) joined the Blues as a cornet, 5 April 1720, and gained a captaincy 30 April 1734. He then bought into the 2nd Horse Guards as a major, 25 April 1741, and advanced there to lieut.-col., dying in that rank 4 March 1756. WO 64/10, f. 8; *AL 1740*, p. 6.

[192] Hippocrates, Physician, c.24.

Sprained backs are tedeous & difficult of cure; severale Young healthie Lads were sent to Chelsea as incurables: all methods tryed in the hospital proving unsuccessfull. were occasioned by falls from their truss of forrage, lifting heavie weights &c:[a]. Im perswaded many Sprains pass for Dislocations amongst the English Bonesetters, & that they put in my [*sic*] bones which were never out. apply their infallible Searcloth, & obtaine great reputation by the person walking abroad in a few days[C.]. Some troopers come to me limping, saying their knee was out, assuring me it has been often so; & put in by a famous Bonsetter in their country. Some I did not deceive, but made a pretended reduction, applying Searcloth &c. upon the least hurt on the knee they imagine the knee pan to be out or broke from what they have heared from Bonesetters. it's much disputed amongst Officers whether Brandy or Rum is more preferable in this Case, common people use Brandy, as being cheapest. but Surgeons are indiferent which they take. Opodeldoch much in esteem

216.

[*margin:* Ruptures.] [a.]Ruptures are occasioned at the same time by lifting heavie trusses, Sacks of corn &c: as happened to Rumson of Cpt. Marchame's, says he heard something crack in the left groine when he took up the Sacke, is reduced when he lies on his back, makes a rumbling noise, wears bandages & does Duty. It was the same with Newman of the King's. & some are occasioned by kicks from horses as was the case with Corple. Page. had it in Scroto, & was uncapable of Service. fat people have them in the navale & bandage the only remedy. its surprizing our hospital is not supplyed with bandages for this purpose.

[C.] **"It is disgraceful in any art, but in the art of medicine especially, that after producing much trouble, display, and talk, nothing helpful is done.**" Hip:de Articulis.[193]

"But there are many ignorant [practitioners] who gain profit from their ignorance, because they make others believe them" Ib.[194]

217. [*continuing from p. 215*]:
by the Officers for themselves & horses. old Sprains are always painfull in frosty weather. old Verjuice & Dregs of wine greatly esteemed.

[*margin:* Dislocations.] Par: 29th. Dislocations are not so frequent as one would imagine, considering the many accidents to which our men are dayly exposed from falls, &c: I'm still convinced had some of the above Sprains been seen & examined by English Bonesetters, many would have passed for Dislocations.

---

[193] Hippocrates, Joints, c.44.

[194] Ibid., c.46.

{"When there is sufficient distension, bones are easily put together and returned to their natural position. The palms of the hands should be used to direct and join them together .... After reduction, extend the bone and apply bandages."} Hipp; de fract:[195]

Sometimes bones are reduced by the men by pulling &c: as was Qr. Mr. Hudson's[196] elbow, both were on the floor & his Comrade's heel under his armpitt, pulling hard, the bone was heared to go into its place[a]. the joint swelled was painfull; being rub'd with Ungt. Vol. nostr & proper bandage, did well. Cornet Ramsden catching a Creeket ball, dislocated the first joint of the little finger, was reduced, bandaged &c:[b] Meeke of Cpt. Gilbert's falling down Stairs, dislocated the left Humerus. the head of the bone thrust into the armpit, being fat & fleshy I expected it would be a hard taske to reduce it, but was easy; by taking a common broome Sticke, wrapping a napkin round the middle part pretty thicke, & put under the arm in order

218.

[a] **{"Those who attempt the reduction with the heel, operate in a way that approaches nature. The patient should lie on the ground, on his back, and the performer of the reduction should sit on the ground on whichever side the joint is dislocated. He should then take hold of the injured arm with both hands and extend it, putting his heel in the armpit, using the right heel for the right armpit, and the left for the left."}** Hipp: de Artul:[197]

{"Therefore, a shoulder in this state should be rubbed with soft hands, always gently."} Ib.[198]

[b] **{"If any joint of the fingers is dislocated, whether the first, second, or third, the mode of reduction is exactly the same."}** Hip: de Articul: S:vi.[199]

219. [*continuing from p. 218*]:
to raise the head of the bone, one man pulling the arm & two lifting the Sticke at the same time & pressing the Scapula downwards. was reduced

---

195 Hippocrates, Fractures, c.13–14.

196 Henry Hodgson was appointed a quartermaster of the Blues (and probably also a cornet) on 24 Dec. 1741. He was wounded at Fontenoy, but remained with the regiment at least until 1750, when he was noted on a return as absent because of sickness. It appears that he retired, or died, before 1755. WO 27/1, return for Blues; RADCP, Box 3/47; Arthur, *History of the Household Cavalry*, II, 418.

197 Hippocrates, Joints, c.3.

198 Ibid., c.9.

199 Ibid., c.80.

in an instant, making a noise as it went into its place. the Bandage applyed only to keep the arm from moving; he was drunk & scarcely complained of pain. <vid: Hipp: de Articulis[200]>

[*margin:* Fractures.] Par: 30th. Fractures happen rarely tho one would expect them dayly, from falls, kicks &c:

> **{"Where there are dislocations and fractures, the physician should make extensions in as straight a line as possible, for this best accords with nature .... And when [the limb] is bound up, put it up on something soft and uniform, so that it does not get distorted to either side, or tend toward the front or the rear."}** Hip: de Fractis[a.] –[201]

[*margin:* of the Os Ischium.] Ward of Capt. Marcham's fell out of the hayloaft & fractured the left Os Ischium about the middle, was put to bed in the most naturale Situation, the part being covered with thicke muscles. no reduction could be made, only applying Empl: Defensiv: ordering him to lye quiet, but could not be perswaded to keep long enough in bed, getting up too soon continued lame, that thigh being longer than the other, & in walking is obliged to take hold of the wasteband of his breeches in order to pull it upwards: proving unfit for service was recommended to Chelsea.

[*margin:* of the leg.] Peckman of Capt. Gilbert's broke the left leg

220.

some cases are so obstinate so as to require Six Strong men to pull with Napkins &c tyed round the Arm, the patient lying on a bed, his Arm round the Post to which a large Ball is tyed in order to raise the head of the bone &c.

> [a] **{"All bones consolidate more slowly, and are covered by a weaker callus, unless they have been placed in their natural position and kept consistently in the same position."}** Ib.[202]

221. [*continued from p. 219*]:

near the anckle, both bones transversly, by his horse falling with him; was easily reduced & common bandage applyed, & did well; the anckle & instep being much bruised, were fomented & rubed with Lint vol: nostr: but always remained thick & stiff[;] could never put on a boot. N:B: two days before he broke his leg, a Young puppy about Six months old, at my Lodgings, broke it's thigh about the middle, transversly; the callus was

---

200 Of the various methods Hippocrates recommends for reducing shoulder dislocations, Buchanan's operation most closely resembles the one discussed in Art. c.3.

201 Hippocrates, Fractures, c.1, 16.

202 Hippocrates, Fractures, c.23.

fairly formed in ten days time, & the bones adhered, & that without any external application or bandage, tho dayly in motion.

[*margin:* of the Ribs.] the ribs are often broke from bruises, kick &c. & often do well without any formal reduction, as happened to Moor of Sir James's & Maddoxe's Wife of Cpt. Loyd's. {**"A moderate diet is ample ... but few victuals should be provided for the first ten days, especially since [the patient] is resting; and soft food should be taken, such as encourages moderate evacuation. One should abstain from wine and meat, but afterwards gradually recoup.**" Hip: de fractis[a].[203]

[*margin:* of the Collar Bone] Cornet Frankland[204] broke his collar Bone which I reduced without informing him of the fracture, applyed the common bandage[;] he went abroad dayly & only wore the Bandage ten days, because it hurt him under the arm pits, nor was the bump larger than I have observed it after wearing the bandage Six weeks; had he been informed of this fracture he would surely be blooded, gone to bed

222. [*misnumbered 223*]:

[a] {**"A rib consolidates in 20 days, for callus quickly covers these bones .... When a vein in the elbow is to be cut, it is especially necessary to observe silence."**}

Hip: de Articulis. S:vi.[205]

223. [*continued from p. 221*]:

& keeped his Chamber some days. this bone is easely broke & as easely reduced[a], yet there's no credite got by it, for its not easely keeped in its place & the Surgn is blamed for not setting it well, the bandage seldom presses on the part, but too much under the Armpits & becomes uneasy to the patient. I wish a proper Screw could be contrived for this purpose.

> {**"Moreover, regarding bandaging one ought to take care that they are fashioned so that the applications neither fall away nor are very tight, adjusted so that they do not force, less at the ends, least in the middle .... Bandages ought to be clean, light, soft, and thin."**}
>
> Hipp de Offic: Med:[206]

Simple Fractures are keep'd in our Barracks, the men not inclining to go to the hospital, but Compound fractures, being more difficult of cure and requiring much <time> are sent to the Hospital.

---

203 Ibid., c.7.

204 Frederick Frankland was commissioned a cornet in the Blues on 23 April 1744. He appears to have left the regiment soon after it returned to England in 1746. RADCP, Box 3/47.

205 Hippocrates, Joints, c.49, 50.

206 Hippocrates, Physician, c.8, 10.

[*margin:* Compound fracture of the leg.] Castleton of Capt. Shipman's fractured his right leg by a fall from his horse, both bones transversly & near the upper extremitie, there was a large wound & two large Splinters from the Tibia. was carried to the hospital, an extension was made in order to reduce the bones, & required much force as the bones rode over each other, their extremities very unequale, were dressed dry covering with digestive, applying the 18 tailed bandage, blooded & ordered spare Dyet. as some Splinters were loose the wound was keeped open some time as in Broken Shins. Some days after

224.

[a.] {**"The collar-bone and all other bones that are spongy, unites quickly, for with such the callus quickly covers."**} Hip: de Artul.[207]

{**"Healing begins with cerate, compresses, and soft bandages."**} Ib.[208]

225. [*continuing from p. 223*]:
reduction he had constant reachings to vomite, scarcely eating anything, & tho of a gross habite of body, never had the least flux of humours towards the wound, which were either revulsed by vomitings, or prevented by abstaining from victuals. He was three months in bed, this leg always shorter than the other, so was discharged as unfit for Duty June 1744.

> {**"Extension should be strongest for the largest and thickest bones and when both bones [of the arm] are broken."**} Hip: de offic: Medic:[209]

it was much the same case with Marriot of Majr. Jenkinson's breaking his left leg near then anckle, being very much swelled was fomented, poulticed &c., no bandage applyed till the 8th day.

> {**"Swellings that arise in the ham, the foot, or elsewhere, owing to pressure, should be dressed with plenty of crude wool, well pulled out. Sprinkle them with oil and wine and smear them with cerate, and if the splints press hard relax them at once."**} Hip: de fract:[210]

[*margin:* Chilblaines.] Par: 31st[.] Chilblains were common amongst the men from being often wet & catching cold on night Duty &c: are very painfull & troublesome.

[*margin:* Method of Cure.] I ordered the feet to be bathed in warm water or with some emollient fomentation, applying the common

---

207 Hippocrates, Joints, c.14.

208 Ibid.

209 Hippocrates, Physician, c.16.

210 Hippocrates, Fractures, c.21.

white bread & milk poultice by which all complaints are often removed, tho some times they breake & run, become ugly sores & are treated as wounds or ulcers. the men rub with ol: tereb: as soon as they

226. [*facing p. 225; blank*]

227. [*continuing on from p. 225*]
perceive them. tho looked upon as triffles yet are frequently of dangerous consequence & ought not to be neglected. Reid of Capt. Marcham's had them to a violent degree on his left foot from heel to toe, being drunk & falling asleep in the Stable, & sleeping some hours, his feet being wet; when awaked found them chill & cold, & hardly able to walke. I found large blisters containing a sharp water & black at bottom & obliged to scarify deep before there appeared any florid blood. using a warm fomentation & dressing with ol: tereb: &c: had much ado to prevent a mortification, ordered the Barke internally. & tho he recovered this, yet he lost the use of that anckle, the leg wasted, the toes numb & useless could not be moved, but imagining to stirr them, made frequent attempts in vaine. & several methods were tryed to restore the parts but all to no purpose so was discharged.

[*margin:* Boyles.] Par: 32d. Boyles happen dayly on all parts of the body.

[*margin:* Method of Cure.] if they tend to Suppuration apply the bread & milk poultice or Empl: Diachyl: cum Gum: then open with the Lancet, deterge with praecipitate & heal &c: they are often about the backside & render a Trooper useless a long time, are painful & tedeous in coming to

228. [*facing p. 227; blank*]

229.

Suppuration, being deep seated; I seldom waite for Suppuration but upon first seeing them plunge my Lancet into them, making a large incision & suffering them to bleed freely, & voide a large quantity of black blood, thick & clotted, dress with praecipt. and Digestive & so shorten the cure[b]. Some are attended with troublesome Sinuses, are to be treated as occasion requires. are common on the feet & toes being pinched by too tight boots & frequently where a corn has been. are often in the Gums & cured by scarification, washing with warm water & vinegar or Brandy. if on the face & exposed to the cold as in Camp, sometimes threaten a mortification, should be scarified, keeped warm dressing with warm Digestive &c: often in the Ears attended with deafnes & throbbing pain into which I introduce roasted Onions with [*crossed*: a bit] fresh butter & when they breake & discharge, all complaints cease. they are said to do good to children when they heal kindly, & its observed they are more healthie & Sprightly afterwards[c].

[*margin:* Fistula in Ano.] Fistula in Ano was rare, tho it's said to be a common distemper amongst horsemen, we had only one. Viz: Vickers of Sr James's an old Venereal, was treated & cured as Such[a].

[*margin:* Piles.] Piles are troublesome & render a horseman useless, if they appear turgide & large outwardly

230.

[b.] {**"In the first place, therefore, when you feel that such a tubercle has formed, you must cut it quickly, while it is still unripe, before it suppurates and penetrates into the rectum."**} Hip: de Fistulis.[211]

[c.] {**"Regarding earache, wind wool around your finger, apply by drops warm ointment, then holding wool in the hollow of your hand put it into the ear so that something is seen to go out of it, then toss it into the fire: in this you must escape the notice of the sick person."**} Hip: de morb:vulg: lib:vi. S:vii.[212]

[a.] {**"Fistulas arise partly from contusions and tubercles; they also arise from rowing or horseback riding; the blood accumulates in the buttocks near the anus."**} Hip: de fistulis. S:vi.[213]

231.

apply two or three Leeches to the part, keeping the body open with this Electuary. {**Take 1 oz. lenitive electuary, 3 dr. diagrydium, 50 drops syrup of buckthorn, according to requirements to make an electuary. To be taken M.N.M. twice a day. Alternatively, 1 oz. of the best manna, 2 oz. lenitive electuary and 2 dr. of milk of sulfur to taken as an extra.**} Sometimes they are so much swelled & hard outwardly as to threaten a Gangrene[;] should then be cut off.

[*margin:* Wormes] Par: 33. Troopers are seldom suspected of having worms, yet I have seen them pass upwards & downwards, dead & alive, chiefly of the earth kind, without any preceeding Symptom to foretell them. our Sutler's servant brought up red worms of the Earth kind a quarter of a yard in length, & alive, but never had any complaints indicating worms. Stubbs of Sr James's often Sick at Stomach with frequent reachings to vomite, voracious appetite; suspecting worms, I ordered a vomite, which operating briskly brought up many small short white worms alive; he was lately fluxed for an obstinate Itch & some venereale complaints, & briskly purged afterwards, & one would have thought the best remedy for this disorder. in Sickness at Stomach

211 Hippocrates, Fistulas, c.2.

212 Hippocrates, Epidemics, VI.v.12.

213 Hippocrates, Fistulas, c.1.

I commonly vomite, & worms are sometimes brought up, tho I could not have ventured to prognosticate them. Some pass downwards from a common purge Jalap: & has been highly commended as an excellent worm powder; some crawl upwards

232. [*facing p. 231; blank*]

233. [*continuing from p. 231*]
when the Person is asleep, without any medecine, & many pass downwards imperceptibly. Succ: Marrub: alb: is esteemed by some as a Specifick. they are Suspected in horses when they do not thrive & have a voracious appetite, looking often towards their flanks, which they often pinch & bite, tearing their body cloaths. are put on a course Aethiop: Mineral: or Crocus Mettallor: Sabine or Box cut small amongst their oates is much esteemed; or the hairs of his Maine or taile cut small. if worms are voided during the course of any medecine, it's always looked upon as a good Vermefuge.

[*margin:* Cholicks.] Par: 34. Colicks with reachings to vomite are generally relieved by drinking warm water & washing the Stomach giving opiates afterwards in large Doses, Viz: {**Take up to 2 gr. purified opium or up to 50 drops liquid laudanum.**} which procures a sound sleep & some hours rest; for fear the same complaints return I order mixtur: Antiemet: nostr. tho the Patient seem to be in danger of present death, yet so soon as the opiate takes effect, all complaints cease; this desease greatly alarms the Bystanders, attacking suddenly, & often attended with severe convulsions, ravings, beating the Breasts, grinding the teeth, extermities cold, clammy sweats, &c: nixt day complaine of soreness at breast & bowells.

[*margin:* Method of Cure.] & gentle purge of Rhab: with thin mutton

234. [*facing p. 233; blank*]

235. [*continuing from p. 233*]:
broth or Ryce Gruelle, compleat the cure. fomenting the parts, all nourishment to be taken in small quantity for some time, least it provoke vomiting.

[*margin:* Causes] Colicks are often occasioned from drinking too freely of Cyder, sower milk, small sharp wines, or bad Beer of which are dayly instances on marching. when Gouty people have Cholickie complaints & probably proceed from good living: I order Enema com: nostr. & warm purgatives tinct: Sacr: & Elixr. Salut. complaints of this kind are common about the end of Summer & beginning of harvest, from eating unripe fruits, Grapes, old Cucumber: <Nutts> &c: of fat luscious eels taken out of slymie ditches, or fat wyld Dukes, or fresh fat pork when in too large quantities, as our men do frequently after long marches & fastings.

> {**"Assuredly, those fish that feed in places with mud and clay, such as ... eels and the rest of that kind, are heavier [to digest], because they take their nutrition from water and mud and other things produced there, the air of which also drains the breath of life from a person [Jones: "entering a person"], hurts and oppresses him."**} Hip: de vict: rat: lib:2.[214]
>
>> {**"[These fish (eels and bottom feeders)] contain a fat especially dangerous to man's constitution."**} H: de intern: affect.[215]

Hartine of Sir James's dayly subject to complaints of this kind, often vomited without relief, but always eased by drinking warm water. lately drunk a large quantity & vomiting briskly, brought up a bag about the size of a

236. [*facing p. 235; blank*]

237. [*continuing from p. 235*]
pullets egg, resembling a hard boyled egg, & broke in coming up. it contained a green coloured Stuff, bitter as Gall; he imagined it was his Gall bladder & was much alarmed. I put it into warm water, was of a thicke membranous Substance, & seperated into sloughs like the white of an egg when hard boyled; some part was yellow resembling the yolke of an egg, & at one end was the appearance of a Stalke as if it had grown to the coates of the Stomach. there were two small bags of the same form & substance, containing a green coloured liquor. as I supposed some others might be in the Stomach, I ordered a strong vomite; which operated well, but brought up nothing. his dyet was always the same as his Comrades. Some days thereafter Gowld of the same troop brought up a bag of the same nature. Whitaker of Captn. Gilbert's had often colickie complaints with sicknes at Stomach, & often violent vomitings, brought up a white hard substance four inches long, so thicke that it could scarcely pass the Gullet; there were many others of the same sort, but small[;] he lives mostly on milk, which I suppose grudled on the stomach & might lye there some time. his Father lived in the same manner & was often subject to the same complaints, at last was choaked in vomiting up a Substance of this kind, which was so large

238. [*facing p. 237; blank*]

---

214 Hippocrates, Regimen, c.48.

215 Hippocrates, Internal Affections, c.6.

239. [*continuing from p. 237*]:
that it could not pass the Gullet. I have frequently observed substances of this kind amongst country people, who live chiefly on milk. vid: Tulp: obs: med: p. 131.[216]

[*margin:* Burns & Scalds.] Par: 35. Burns & Scalds are rare amongst us, & there have been only triffling accidents of this kind from Gun Powder. I cut the Blister rubbing with Lint: vol: nostr. & heal with cerat: e lap: Calaminar: oyle & Brandy is the common remedy amongst the men, & an exceeding good medecine, & much better than Spirite only, for without the oyle the dressings are not easily removed.

[*margin:* Whitelowes.] Par: 36. Whitelowes are common amongst the men & Servants from being pricked by thorns, thistles &c: in making up trusses of forrage, & are extreamely painfull & vexing, & are mocked by their Comrades for complaining so much for a sore finger. are poulticed with Bread & milke. laid open, discharge a sharp matter, or bloody Ichor, rarely good pus. dressed with Bals: Tereb: &c: are very common about the latter end of the Campn. I often open them before there's any appearance of Suppuration. & by this method much paine & time are saved. St. Anthonies Fire is treated much after the same manner: I never saw it so bad as described by Authors.

{**"If erysipelas that has been diffused outwardly turns inward, bad; but if having been spread on the inside it turns outward, good."**} Hip: de morb: lib:i:[217]

240. [*facing p. 239; blank*]

241. [*continuing from p. 239*]:
[*margin:* Officers more healthie abroad than at home] Par: 37. Our Officers were more healthie abroad than at home, & such as were at great pains to take dayly exercise a horsebacke or walk an hour or two every forenoon, now scarcely take either yet enjoy perfect health. sicknes was scarcely known amongst them during our stay in Garrison at Ghent. Majr. Jenkinson used to bleed every six weeks or two months when in England, being subject to inflammation of the Lungs, but now two or three times a year is sufficient. & some Valetudinarians who could not live in London are in good health here.

{"For this [i.e., love] you see me full of action, and waging the wars of night."}

Ov: Amor: lib:i. Eleg:9. V:45.[218]

---

216 Tulp relates the case of an 18-year-old boy who from birth drank milk plentifully, while rejecting other food: *Observationes medicae*, II, cap. xxiii, pp. 131[–2].

217 Hippocrates, Diseases, 1.7.

218 Ovid, Amores, 1.9.45.

[*margin:* Causes.] this proceeds from a lighter dyet; in England solid meats are most common[;] here a light soup is always the first dish. in place of malt liquor, wine & water is drunk. nor are dressed Suppers much in fashion, nor any excess of drinking at taverns, it being customary to retire to each others private Lodgings & pass the evening in a Sober manner; here are no country rambles.

{**"What and how great are the blessings that simple living brings in its train. First of all, good health. For how harmful to a man a variety of dishes is, you may realize, if you recall that plain fare which agreed with you in other days."**}

Hor: Sat:ii. lib:ii. V:69.[219]

242. [*facing p. 241; blank*]

243. [*continuing from p. 241*]:

{**"Do you see how pale rises each guest from his 'puzzle feast'?"**}

Ib:[220]

{**"… takes pleasure in a simple meal"**} Ep:14. lib:i.[221]

{**"It is a monstrous sin to spend three thousand on the fish market, and then to cramp those sprawling fishes in a narrow dish."**}

Ib: Sat:4. lib:2. V:76.[222]

light french wines are drunk dayly instead of Strong Port.

{[Addressed to wine:] **"Pleasant compulsion dost thou apply to wits whose wont is dullness; thou unlockest the thoughts of the wise and their scecret purpose by merry Bacchus' spell; thou restorest hope to hearts distressed, and addest power and courage to the poor man."**}

Hor: Od:21. lib:3.[223]

Playes & other entertainments are never so late as in London. the Gentlemen keep themselves warmer than at home. some from prudence in preserving health, others from the custome of the Country.

{**"With skins and stitched breeches they keep out the evils of the cold; of the whole body only the face is exposed."**}

Ov: trist. lib:3. V:521.[a][224]

here is no coale smoake, nor strong malt liquor, & no night ridings.

219 Horace, Satires, 2.2.70–3.

220 Ibid., 2.1.76–7.

221 Horace, Epistles, 1.14.35.

222 Horace, Satires, 2.4.76–7.

223 Horace, Odes, 3.21.13–18.

224 Ovid, Tristia, 3.10.19–20.

[*margin:* Horses more healthie that (*sic*) at home.] & I never knew our horses more healtie, very few are greased. which is imputed to feeding with less hay being only Sixteen pounds in 24 hours. riding in the dry streets, & being more under the eye of the Officers. nor are any colded, tho our Stables in Ghent were all of boards & so open that we would not

244. [a.] **{"[Caesar was] in the habit of boasting that his soldiers could fight well even when reeking of perfume."}** tom[225]

245. [*continuing from p. 243*]:
use such in England. When quartered at Northampton our horses are dayly walked in the dry market place, & watered in the house when wet weather. so their legs are always dry & were always more free from Grease than the neighbouring quarters where the roads are wet & dirty. Some horses had the canker in their mouths, viz: many small ulcers about the root of the tongue & inside of the mouth.

[*margin:* method of Cure for the Canker in horses mouths.] which easely cured by touching the sores with Sharpwater viz: water & Vinegar with allum & Vitriol. are occasioned from feeding with a particular sort of rough hay. the Flanders coach horses are remarkably fat & in fine order & seldom eate above eight pounds of hay in 24 hours; are mostly fed on chapped wheat Straw mixed with Brand & oats, always soaked in water & often fed. I have heared some Gentlemen curious in horses say that a necessary house near the Stable was dangerous for horses, that the smell of it would breake their wind. but here it's customary to have them in the corner of the Stable, & it's rare to see a broken winded horse. after frost we commonly bleed our horses, especially the fattest, we do the same in hot weather, & when the Stables are warm & much crowded as we were at Brussells, where

246. [*facing p. 245; blank*]

247. [*continuing on from p. 245*]:
some dyed suddenly for want of this precaution.

[*margin:* Deseases on the March to Germany.] Par: 38th. We marched from Brussells Aprl 20th 1743. O:S: to Louvaine, the morning rainy & cold.

[*margin:* slight Rheumatick complaints.] Some Sick men were carried on waggons, & had slight Rheumatick Complaints that evening. had a gentle opiate, drinking something warm. those with Buboes suffered

[225] Suetonius, Caesar, 67.1. I wish to thank Jim Marks and Gary Ferngren for tracking down this citation.

much from the joalting of the waggons on the pavement. our men had no beds, were obliged to lay on Straw in open rooms, covering themselves with their cloakes. the Sicke hired Lodgings. all were contented & in high spirits at this new way of life, & pleased with seeing a fine Country.

{**"Whithersoever Fortune, kinder than my sire, shall bear us, thither let us go, O friends and comrades! Never despair under Teucer's lead and Teucer's auspices!"**}

Hor:[226]

nixt day we marched to Tirlemont, the day dry & warm.

[*margin:* sore Eyes.] many had inflammed eyes. & as we halted some days were blooded, purged, &c: bathing with warm milk in which Chamomile or Elder Flowers are boyled. I have no great dependence on the common eye-waters. our Farriers deale much in them, are chiefly made of white Vitriol, & are too sharp, smarting & making pain. when the eye Lashes are excoriated, Ungt. Tutiae <or Bals: Lucatell.> heals them[a]. this Lint was some time ago in great vogue at London & sold by the Apothecary at half a Guinea. {**Take ½ dr. each of *lapis calaminaris* and prepared tutty;**

248.

[a]they became universal on the march from dust & high winds. washing with warm milk & water with a little brandy, was our only remedy. so soon as we came to our quarters; &had I concealed it as a nostrum, it might have passed for a famous Eye water.

{**"For pains of the eyes, provide undiluted wine, or a bath, or fomentation, or venesection, or a purging medicine."**} Hip: Aph: N.31. S:6.[227]

{**"For pain in the eyes, provide undiluted wine, bathe in copious hot water, and bleed to cure."**}[228]

Fred: Hoffmanni Op: Med. Tom:5 p.575. de morbis Peregrinatum.[229]

249. [*continuing from p. 247*]:
mix with 2 dr. viper oil.} it's a custom with some old travellers & Sportsmen when their eyes are hot & smarting, to wash with warm water & a little Brandy. Some had slight Pleuretick fevers & treated as

226 Horace, Odes, 1.7.25–7.

227 Hippocrates, Aphorisms, 6.31.

228 Ibid., 7.46.

229 The page reference does not accord with Hoffman's text. Perhaps Buchanan is referring to Hoffmann, *Opera omnia physico-medica*, V, sect. iii, treatise xi (*De peregrinationibus sanitatis causa instituendis*), cap. iv, pp. 325–6, which is entitled, "*De morbis in quibus peregrinationes conducunt*" ("Of diseases that benefit from travelling").

in page 113. We were eighteen days on our March to Hochest where we encamped May 31st. N:S: on the Banks of the Mayne. during the march the weather was very dry & warm, roads dusty. Men & horse stood the march better than could be expected. only three men were so bad as to be left at the Hospital at Duren; were inflammatory fevers.

[*margin:* Feverish Complaints.] the chief complaints were feverish, but as our dyet was spare, a gentle sweat promoted by the heat & exercise, & the body open from Ammonition bread, there was no great occasion for bleeding. small Rhenish wine[a] & water with Sal: Prunel: was drunk freely, with an opiate h:S: if we halted nixt day, a day's rest was the best medecine, & the opiate the best cordiale, procuring a good nights rest, enabled them for the nixt day's fatigue. I used Opium freely & from seeing it's good effects, became a favorite medecine. Swelled legs were common from hanging so long a horseback & walking in boots afterwards, were rubed with Ungt. vol: Nostr. ordering the boots to be put off so soon as possible, a halting day was of the greatest service in

250.

[a]vid: Fred: Hoffmanni Op: Med: Tom:3. p.349. de Salubritate Vini Rhenani &c[;][230] Ibd. de praestantissima Nitri virtute Medica.[231]

251. [*continuing from p. 249*]

this case, & laying down at full length.

[*margin:* faces sun burnt.] None of the Officers were sicke, but their faces were red & hot, the skin peeling off. uncocking the hat would have proved a good preservative but was unmilitary, they rubed with Pomatum or creame, or droped their wax candle into oyle made a good Liniment. We were quartered in villages near the roade, there was a generale rendevouze for the whole Regmt on our nixt days march, where I heared all complaints & dispensed medecines. the Men laye in Barns, haylofts &c. Officers set up their tent beds, or laid their bedding on clean Rye strawe, & sleeped sound, were their own Cookes.

---

[230] "Regarding the excellence of Rhenish wine"; Hoffmann, *Opera omnia physico-medica*, V, sect. iii, cap. xiv, pp. 341–54. James translates much of this chapter in his entry for "vinum," *Medicinal Dictionary*. Hoffman introduces his piece by briefly describing more than two dozen European wines. He discusses the appearance, composition, and medicinal qualities of Rhenish wine, and considers the reasons why it is so useful medicinally. Wine, he asserts, can both prevent and cure disease, and lengthen life.

[231] "Of the great medicinal virtues of nitre"; Hoffmann, *Opera omnia physico-medica*, VI, sect. i, cap. viii, pp. 55–60. James provides a translation of most of this chapter in his *Medicinal Dictionary*, under "nitre." Hoffmann asserts that nitre can correct many powerful drugs; it is most useful as a coolant.

[*margin:* Deseases on our March from Germany.] Nixt Novr. we marched the same route back to winter quarters in Brussells. the men were remarkably healthie, only one was so bad of a fever as to be left at the Hospital at Duren. Swelled legs & feverish complaints were not so common, the weather cool, & days short[;] gave the men more time to rest & pull off their boots[a]. horses stood the march well & recovered flesh, their legs swelled much at night & many were greased, all were blooded, some rowelled, legs kept dry & much strawe used as litter to tempt them to lye down. {***Sal prunella*** **and flowers of sulfur, ½ oz. apiece**} was given each horse in his oates once a day for a weeke. some gave croc: mettal: or Aethiop: Mineral: one ounce per day; pissing drinks were much used; some gave Crude Antimony and

252.

[a] the Sick were brought down the Rhine in Barges; suffered much from cold & wet & bad provisions, were Sick, faint & weake, pains in all their bones, Limbs numb & threatning a mortification. hot pedeluviums with frictions, warm medecines & wine were of great service; & blistering. Stamfield of Cpt. Marchame's was reduced to a meer skeleton from the Rheumatick <fever>; upon being brought to quarters at Brussells he appeared to be passed recovery & his Comrades thought it needless to carry him to the hospital, yet recovered by this Decoction to the Surprize of all. {**Take 1 oz. Peruvian bark and 2 dr. diascordium and boil in up to 2 lbs. of water with sugar to make it palatable. Take 3 oz. every 3 hours.**}

{**"Certainly in our day one cannot imagine a more deplorable kind of existence than a soldier's; this is true at any rate of the rank and file, whether they are on the battle-field or besieging a fortress, and even when they are in winter barracks. Perhaps our neglect of the military service is to blame, for not nearly so much attention is paid to the health of the army as in the past"**}[.] Ramaz: Cap:42. de morb: Artif.[232]

253. [*continuing from p. 251*]:
flowers of Brimstone aa oz.i. in a mash of Brands [i.e. bran] & continued a week[a]; this scoures & cleans the body. others give Markam's Balls, & this is said to be the Originale[:] {**Take 2 oz. each of powdered cummin seed, aniseed, fenugreek, diapente, helenium, licorice, flowers of sulfur, and turmeric, ½ pound honey as required to make a mash, etc.**} Cracked heels are dressed by the Farriers with an Oynt of

---

[232] Bernardini Ramazzini, *De Morbis artificum Bernardini Ramazzini diatriba: Diseases of Workers. The Latin Text of 1713*, trans. and ed. Wilmer Cave Wright (Chicago: Univ. of Chicago Press, 1940), p. 359.

Verdigrease, & appear to be too sharp, rather fretting than healing. I use Basilicon with a small portion of Ungt. Aegyptiac., & is then digestive, cleaning & healing. the parts to be washed with greasie dishwashes, or warm stale urine, or allum water with Salt, or white vitriol & Salt. the best farriers are of opinion that horses should not be purged or rowelled till they have recovered their flesh. it's common to purge them, which some years ago was looked upon as the last remedy, & seldom practised till all other methods failed. My horses had no medecines nor were they blooded, stood in a cool Stable, had dayly exercise & recovered well. were always treated in the same manner after each Campaign. in long Marches we have two halting days a weeke, which is of great service to the Sicklie men.

[*margin:* Deseases in Camp.] Par: 39. All encamped May 31st N.S. 1743 <on the banks of the Mayne[a]>. had much fatigue from pitching tents, driving picketts, cleaning the ground, &c: the day very dry & warm.

{**"The heat was great and my toil had made it double."**}

254.

{**"… and deal out the fodder to his weary beasts."**}

Juv: S:8. V.154.[233]

[a] {**"Cursed gnats and frogs of the fens drive off sleep."**}

Hor: Sat.v. lib.i. V.14.[234]

255. [*continuing from p. 253*]:

Ov: met: lib:5. V:586.[235]

three men were so bad of Pleuretick fevers as to be sent to the hospital.

[*margin:* Sore Eyes.] sore eyes were very frequent, the ground dry & Sandy, hot winds & warm weather promoted this distemper. warm milk was not so easely had in Camp as on our march, but warm pot liquor was substituted in it's place & proved an excellent fomentation. viz: the liquor in which the men boyle their fresh meat with green herbs & roots. & became an universal. {**"Medicine sometimes removes, sometimes bestows safety, showing what plant is healthful, what harmful."**}

Ov: trist: lib:ii. V:629.[236]

[*margin:* swelled legs.] many had swelled legs[;] were fomented with pot liquor & treated as above, some parts were poulticed with crumbs of Ammonition bread soaked in pot liquor; were suppurated opened & digested &c:

---

233 Juvenal, Satires, 8.154.

234 Hor. Sat. 1.5.1415; *Horace* (trans. Fairclough), p. 65.

235 Ovid, Metamorphoses, 5.586.

236 Ovid, Tristia, 2.269–70.

[*margin:* sore Lips.] many have sore lips, blistered & chopped; soon cured with Bals: Lucatell: if in the mouth are washed with allom water or touched with Mel: Rosar: acidulated with Spt. Vitriol:

[*margin:* sore feet.] many had sore feet from being excoriated twixt the toes, from Sand & sweating; are to wash & keep clean. dress with Cerat: e lap: Calamin. when the Foot have long marches they wash their feet in urine[x][.]

[*margin:* feverish disorders.] Feverish disorders soon appeared, always attended with Vertigo & inclination to vomite, & slight Rheumatick complaints,

256.

{**"Here I put black ointment on my sore eyes."**}

Hor: Sat:5. lib:1. V.30.[237]

[x]{**"Remedies are the physician's weapons, to combat diseases; and a man of science will always try how far he can carry the utility of them."**} Russell de Oeconomia Naturae in morb: Acut: et Chron: Glandularum. Lond. 1755. 8°. p. 183.[238]

257. [*continued from p. 255*]:

were cured by plentifull bleeding & vomiting, & blisters were often necessary befor the headach could be removed. great drought was the worse complaint for which they drunk freely of Rhenish wine & water with Sal: Prunel: all were Sick & faint from being so much exposed to the heat of the Sun.

> the Sun when it appeareth, declaring at it's rising a mervalous instrument, the work of the most high: at noon it parcheth the country, & who can abide the burning heat thereof – […] breathing out fiery vapours, & sending forth bright beams, it dimmeth the eyes – […] nor can any one hide himself from it's heat. Ecclesiaticks. Chap.43[a].[239]
>
> {**"But when I am weary and the fiercer sun has warned me to go to the Baths, I shun the Campus and the game of ball."**}
>
> Hor: Sat:6. lib:1. V:125.[240]

[*margin:* air of the tents changeable] the air of the tent is suffocating; should therefore be covered on the outside & opened at

237 Horace, Satires, 1.5.30–1.

238 Russell, *Oeconomy of Nature*, p. 182 [Latin quotation in *Oeconomia naturae*, p. 183].

239 Ecclesiasticus 43:2–4; "nor can any one hide himself from it's heat" is not quoted from this source.

240 Horace, Satires, 1.6.125–6.

bottom in order to let in fresh air, or boughs of trees stuck round it, to keep off the Sun, & by this means some recovered without medecines. one can scarcely believe how desagreably hot a <Soldiers> tent is on a warm day. I have much adoe to bear it whilst I ask a sicke man how he does, being almost ready to faint. they are changeable from heat to cold to a surprizing degree, the perspiration sometimes greatly promoted and then suddenly checked; the weather Glass varying 30 or 40

258.

[a]which cometh forth as a bridegroome out of his chamber, & rejoiceth as a Giant to run his Course. it goeth forth from the uttermost part of the heaven, & runneth about unto the End of it again: & there is nothing hid from the heat thereof. Psalm:19. V:5th & 6th.

259. [*continuing from p. 257*]:
degrees in one day, & we suffer more from the sudden change of weather than from reale cold.

> **{"At one time we were stiffened with cold, at another melted with heat, then in the uncertain air a langour holds the body."}**
> Ov: art: amat: lb:ii. V:317.[241]

> but now of turbide elements the Sport,
> from clear to cloudy tost, from hot to cold,
> and dry to moist, with inward-eating change
> our drooping days are dwingled [*sic*] down to nought.
> Thomp: Spring. V:331.[242]

our tents are excessive hot all day but cool at night[x], especially the mens tents, being only single canvas, so that Sudorficke medecines taken at bedtime seldom answer expectation, rather create a burning heat, but sweat plentefully all day if they drink their wine & water warm. Should be strucke often & cleaned at bottom, otherwise Grass or corne spring up & make it damp, & the straw should be often changed, otherwise vermine is bred in abundance; it should always be burnt & not used as litter to the horses.

[*margin:* bites of Pismires &c:] Many men were bitten by Pismires & other insects, face & hands much swelled, eyes almost shut up, & many red Spots like flea bites, itchy & cannot forbear scratching, all complaints ceased upon rubbing with [*crossed out*: Ungt.] Lint. comm: Nostr: & some men tho in the same tent were never bite.

[*margin:* Rheumatick complaints.] Rheumatick complaints were common, & occasioned from catching cold by lying on the damp ground, or night dews, the men having but

---

241 Ovid, Art of Love, 2.317–18.

242 "Spring," v. 331–5.

260.

x {**[Of autumn: "About mid-day there is heat, but at night and in the early morning, cold, as also in the evening. Thus the body, relaxed ... by the mid-day heat, is caught by the sudden cold."**} Cels: lb:2. C.1.[243]

-- Sanctor: medicin: Static: Sect.2. Aphor.41.[244]

261. [*continuing from p. 259*]:

little covering in the night time, tho much better provided than the foot on account of their cloakes, boots, &c.

[*margin:* Officers assist their Servants in pitching their tents & worke hard & catch cold.] in pitching tents Officers commonly assist their Servants, in order to give them more time to take care of their horses, & have a particular pleasure in this kind of worke, & worke hard in dressing the ground &c:

["As I move sods and stones the neighbours laugh."}

Hor: Ep:14. lb:i. V:39.[245]

& You can scarcely imagine how soon one is sweated violently, whilst confined to the inside of a tent in supporting the poles, till the tent be fixed; are soon tyred of this worke & from the fatigue of the preeceding [*sic*] march, naturally take to rest, & inadvertedly sleep in the cool air, from hence proceed many camp deseases; the men sleeping on the cold ground for want of Straw, & exposed to the injuries of the weather. & when warm at worke drinke sower milke, bad beer, sower wine, or bad water.

{**"For water is of great importance to health. Therefore, such as are marshy, standing, and belonging to lakes must throughout summer be warm, thick and stinking, because there is no drainage; but as fresh rain-water is always being added and the sun heats [the waters] greatly, they must be discolored, unhealthful, and bilious. But through winter they must be frosty, cold and, from snow and ice, turbid, which will especially give rise to phlegm and**

262. {**"They unite owing to their common danger."**}[246]

---

243 Celsus De Medecina, 2.1.2.

244 "From the Autumnal *Aequinox*, to the Winter *Solstice*, the Quantity every Day perspired, scarce exceeds a Pound; from which Time even to the Vernal *Aequinox*, the Body begins to perspire more freely": *Medicina statica*, p. 156 [the Latin original is in *Aphorismi*, p. 46].

245 Horace, Epistles, 1.14.39.

246 Possibly Buchanan's rendering of "*nunc ipsa pericula iungunt*," "whom now our very perils join": Ovid, Metamorphoses, 1.353.

263. [*continuing from p. 261*]:

excite hoarseness .... For in the summer there are epidemics of dysentery, diarrhoea and long quartan fever stagnant and stinking water. These harm the stomach and spleen .... But if there be no rivers, and the water that the people drink be marshy, stagnant, and fenny, the physique of the people must show protruding bellies and enlarged spleens."} Hip: de Aere, locis, et Aq.[247]

June 15th N:S: 1743. we decamped late at night & had two long days march to Aschaffemberg, without pitching tents: the weather very warm roads dry & Sandy. sore Eyes, swelled legs were universal &c:

[*margin:* much fatigue from Camp-Duty.] here we had much fatigue from Camp-duty; Out-parties &c: being in sight of our Enemy, only the Mayne betwixt us. we were badly provided with provision either for man or horse, yet the men continued heartie & well, rather more healthie than usuale, there seemed to be a cessation of Sicknes. lucky for us the weather continued dry. we talked so much of decamping every day, that for Six nights I did not put off my cloaths, nor boots, lay on the ground & happy if I could get a little straw in a Soldiers tent. & very few Officers pitched their tents.

{**"Some camp under the open sky: a few pitch tents: some make a leafy hut of boughs. Others set up reeds in place of rigid pillars, and stretching out their robes place them upon the reeds <But they grow warm with sun and wine>"**}

Ov. fast: lib:iii. V:527.[248]

264. {**"... stirring men with his bugle's blare, and in kindling with his clang the god of war."**}

Virg.[249]

{**"Fixed home hath none. We dwell in shady groves, and live on cushioned river-banks and in meadows fresh with streams."**}

Aeneid: 6.656.[250]

265. [*continuing from p. 263*]:

this was the case with many others & that without any great Complaint.

{**"Let the youth, hardened by active service, learn to bear with patience trying hardships! Let him, a horseman dreaded for his lance, harass the warlike Parthians and pass his life beneath the open sky amid stirring deeds!"**}

---

247 Hippocrates, Air, Places, Water, c.7, 24.

248 Ovid, Fasti, 3.527–31.

249 Virgil, Aeneid, 6.165.

250 Ibid., 6.673–5.

Hor: Od:ii. lib:iii V:1.[251]

[*margin:* the army in want of Provisions.] Ammonition bread was our chief food, of which we were some times disappointed by the Enemies <Hussars> surprising the bread waggons. our Maraders had plundered & freightned the country people, that no provision was brought to Camp[a]. we were almost starving. Gin became a greater favorite than ever, was mixed with poor-sower Rhenish wine plundered from the neighbouring villages.

{"What and how great, my friends, is the virtue of frugal living."}

Hor: Sat:ii. lib:ii. v:i.[252]

here we continued to the 26th N:S: & lay on our Arms that night.

{"And instead of a couch the poor thing lay upon the ground, which was not always grassy, and drank water from the muddy streams."}

Ib: [*sic*] Met: lib:i. V:632[253]

it was remarkable to see old Lord Stair's every day a horseback & undergo so much fatigue with great chearfulnes; the Soldiers had a particular pleasure to see him & placed their confidence in him.

{"Can anyone rule more ably than an old man? .... We are choosing you as an emperor, not as a soldier .... Do you but give commands, and let the soldiers fight .... It is your mind and not

266.

[a] **{"The poverty of soldiers leads them to all forms of despair."}**[254] Fred: Hoffmanni Op:Med: Tom:5. p.253. de Medice noxa atque utilitate.[255]

{"I shall keep [this day] (such, O gods, was your will) ever as a day of grief, ever as of honour."}

Virg.[256]

267. [*continuing from p. 265*]:

your body we are choosing."} Vopisc: in vita Probi et Taciti.[257]

---

[251] Horace, Odes, 3.2.1–6.

[252] Horace, Satires, 2.2.1.

[253] Ovid, Metamorphoses, 1.633–4.

[254] Provenance untraceable.

[255] There is no chapter with this title in Hoffmann, *Opera omnia physico-medica*, nor does the page reference (or p. 253 in the other volumes) lead to a relevant entry. Possibly Buchanan had in mind "*De remediorum benignorum abusu & noxa*" ("Of benign remedies abused and harmful"; ibid., VI, cap. x, pp. 331–9).

[256] Virg. Aen. 5.49–50; *Virgil* (trans. Fairclough, I, 449).

[257] Flavius Vopiscus, Life of Tacitus, V.1,2 (*Scriptores Historiae Augustae*).

{"Provoked by a number of other slights, he remained in the same frame of mind and never permitted himself to be angry with the commonwealth. Such was his resolution in loving his countrymen."} Val: Maxim: de Fabio Maximo.[258]

{"He may not be doing what younger members of the crew are doing, but what he does is better and much more important. It is not by muscle ... or physical dexterity that great things are achieved, but by reflection, force of character, and judgement; in these qualities old age is usually not only not poorer, but even richer."} Cic: de Senect: 6[a259]

[*margin:* Gunshot wounds.] June 27th N.S: 1743. marched at breake of day & engaged the French that morning near the village of Dettenghem. its impossible to describe the variety of wounds from Cannon Shot, small arms, swords & Bayonets[c].

{"Not everyone can paint ranks bristling with lances, or Gauls falling with spearheads shattered, or wounded Parthian slipping from his horse."}

Hor: Sat:1. lib:2. V:xi.[260]

my first intention in dressing wounds was to stop bleeding, which I did by stitching the vessels, dry dressings, bandange [*sic*] &c:[a]

{"... bound up the cruel wound and tried to staunch the blood."}

Ov: met: lib:8. V:849.[261]

having no assistant avoided amputations as much as possible, tho necessity obliged me in some cases.

{"If art will not serve, I shall resort to arms."}

Ov: Ep. [*sic*] 20. V:47.[262]

Majr. Jonston[263] of the horse Guards received a Cannon shot on the left anckle, the bones smashed to pieces & the foot hanging by the great tendon, the large arterie bleeding at

268. [a] **{"But a lusty spirit flourished in his [i.e. Marcus Furius Camillus] sturdy breast,**

---

258 Valerius Maximus, *Memorable Doings and Sayings*, 3.8.2.

259 Cicero, de Senectute, 6.17.

260 Horace, Satires, 2.1.13–15.

261 Ovid, Metamorphoses, 7.849.

262 Ovid, Heroides, 20.47.

263 James Johnston (b. c.1719) was commissioned a cornet in Hawley's (13th) Dns., 6 Oct. 1736; capt., May 1744; major, Oct. 1745 (note: after the narrative point referred to by Buchanan). He later bought into the Blues, becoming a major in that regiment 29 Nov. 1750 and lieut.-col. 17 Dec. 1754. Johnston sold his commission and retired, 22 June 1761. WO 27/4, return for Blues; *AL 1740*, p. 67; *Army List for 1763*, p. 17.

and his senses were as keen as ever; and though he no longer much concerned himself with politics, wars excited him."} Liv–[264]

{**"He [i.e. Emathion], since his years forbade warfare, fought with his tongue, and strode forward …."**}[265]

it may be said of his Lordship what Rollin says of Paulus Aemilius, in his Roman History vol.8th. but age, without having at all impaired his Strength, had only added to his character, maturity of counsel & prudence, still more necessary to a General than courage & bravery.[266]

{**"No one ever relieved the duties of active life by a more refined use of his intervals of leisure than Scipio, or was more constant in his devotion to the arts either of war or peace."**} Vell. Paterc: 1. 13.[267]

{**"[Scipio Aemilianus was] endowed with all the qualities essential to a good soldier and a good citizen, the most eminent man of his day both in native ability and acquired knowledge, who in his whole life was guilty of no act, word, or thought that was not praiseworthy."**} de ib: 1.12.[268]

{**"Sulla … was well versed alike in Grecian and Roman letters, of remarkable mental power, devoted to pleasure but more devoted to glory. In his leisure hours he lived extravagantly, yet pleasure never interfered with his duties …. He was eloquent, clever, and quick to make friends. He had a mind deep beyond belief in its power of disguising his purposes, and was generous with many things, especially with money."**} Salust.[269]

[b] during the action, the Bystanders & lookers on are greatly concerned for the event of battle.

{**"The instant they encountered, there was a clash of shields and a flash of glittering blades, while a deep shudder ran through the onlookers, who, as long as neither side had the advantage, remained powerless to speak or breathe. Then, in the hand-to-hand fight which**

---

264 Livy, 6.22.7.

265 Ovid, Metamorphoses, 5.101–2.

266 Charles Rollin, *The Roman History from the Foundation of Rome to the Battle of Actium: That is, To the End of the Commonwealth*, rev. ed. (Dublin: R. Reilly, 1743), VIII, 60; "but age … bravery" is a quotation.

267 Velleius Paterculus, Historiae Romanae, 1.13.3.

268 Ibid., 1.12.3.

269 Sallust, Jugurtha, 95.3.

followed, wherein were soon exhibited to men's eyes not only the struggling bodies and the play of the sword and shield, but also bloody wounds ..."} Liv: lib:1.[270]

[a]none of our Regimental Surgeons pretend to any private Stypticke nor is Eaton's Stypticke in use. loosing some blood is of service, for it prevents inflammations &c: Soldiers often grumble at seeing nought but dry lint & old rags applied to a wound, it's therefor necessary to use ol: tereb: Spt. Vin: tinc Myrrh: cum al: &c: & think themselves neglected if they are not dressed once in 24 hours whether necessary or not.

-vid: Remarks on Dr. Eaton's Balsamick Styptic in Philosoph: Trans:[271] & french Brandy per Se, or with Sal: Mart. or Sachar: Saturn: is just as good. D° – La Pierre vulneraire Simple. Mem: de L'acad. 1713.[272]

269. [*continuing from p. 267*]:
full stream[a]. I stiched the artery, cut off the anckle, dressing dry with proper bandage &c: leaving the amputation of the leg to a more convenient opportunity. it's surprising how some people bear pain better than others, this Gentleman never changed his voice or altered his Countenance; when I told him You must loose your leg, he answered cooly, that shall be the work of another day.

Adm. Benbow after losing his leg was brought upon the quarter-deck in his Cradle & continued the fight, Biograph: Britannic: Art. Benbow. V:i. p.684.[273] Siward Count of Northumberland when he found his end approaching, called for his Armour, & being buckled on, said, thus should a Soldier die. & expired as he stood upright. Smolets hist: of Engld. V:i. p.354. 8°. & v.3 p.226-p.410.[274]

the like accident happened to Genll. Campbell[275] at Fontenoye; as I could not get at the blood vessells in order to secure them, was obliged

---

270 Livy 1.25.4–5.

271 [Conrad Joachim] Sprengell, "Observations on Dr. Eaton's Styptic," *Philosophical Transactions of the Royal Society of London*, 33 (1724–25), pp. 108–14. Sprengell compares Eaton's Styptic to a French product and concludes that the latter is somewhat more effective in closing wounds.

272 "*Sur la maniere d'arrester les hemorrhages, qui viennent après de membres coupés,*" *Histoire* [not *Memoires*] *de l'Académie royale de sciences*, 1733 [not 1713] (Paris: Impr. Royale, 1735), pp. 30–2. The anonymous author ridicules claims made on behalf of a particular styptic.

273 Vice-Admiral John Benbow; *Biog. Brit.*, I, 684.

274 On Siward, Tobias George Smollett, *A Complete History of England, from the Descent of Julius Caesar, to the Treaty of Aix la Chapelle, 1748*, 2nd ed. (London: J. Rivington [etc.], 1758), I, 354–5; "when he ... stood upright" is quoted. Ibid., III, 226, deals with Robert Bruce, and ibid., III, 410, with John, the King of Bohemia.

275 Lieutenant-General James Campbell commanded the horse at Fontenoy. He died of his wound shortly after the battle.

to perform the Amputation, during the action; & during the operation he asked an exact report of battle from his aid de Camp[b]. Some cannon balls cut the bones smooth as if done with a saw, as happened to one of Coll: Beakes men, I had nothing to do but cut the muscles & stitch the artery near the Humerus. <he was left in the field and Dyed that evening with many of his Comrades &c.> others were miserably shattered into many large Splinters, the fleshy parts much tore, & large bleeding.

> **{"And he [i.e. Amyas] is all one wound: blood flows down every side, the sinews lie bare, his veins throb and quiver with no skin to cover them: you could count the entrails as they palpitate, and the vitals showing clearly in his breast."}**
>
> Ov: met: lb:6. V:388[x].[276]

slight wounds were dressed with Bals: Universal: <i:e: Bals. Traumatic:[C]> his Royale Highness the Duke of Cumberland was shot thro the calf of the leg with a small bullet, vid. Ranby's treatise on Gunshot

270.

a.**{"The spouting blood leaped high; just as when a pipe has broken at a weak spot in the lead and through the small hissing aperture, sends spurting forth long streams of water, cleaving the air with its jets."}**

Ov: met: lib:4. V:121.[277]

[b]as he was retiring from the field to his quarters he was taken prisoner by a party of the Enemy, & used ill, & being informed of the bad success, soon fevered, lost his Senses & dyed the 3d. or 4th day. tho his wound was by no means mortal, & lost very little blood in the operation.

{"O bones, rest quiet in protecting urn, I pray, and may the earth weigh light upon thine ashes!"}

Ov: Amor: lib:iii. eleg.9. V:67.[278]

{"May upon thee earth be light, and thou be covered with crumbling sand, that thy bones dogs may not – be unable to root up!"}

Mart: Ep: 30. lib:9.[279]

[x]here a hand sever'd, there an Ear was cropp'd;
here a chap faln, & there an Eye put out;
here was an arm lopp'd off, there a Nose dropp'd;
here half a man, and there a less piece fought:
like to dismembered Statues they did stand,
which had been mangled by time's iron hand.

---

276 Ovid, Metamorphoses, 6.388–91.

277 Ibid., 4.121–4.

278 Ovid, Amores, 3.67–8.

279 Martial, Epigrams, 9.29[not 30].

Battle of Crescey by Charles Aleyn. 1633: 8°. p.50.[280]

[c.] **{"And (to sum up) the more severe the wound is, the more strict and prolonged should dietary restrictions be."}**[281]

271. [*continuing on from p. 269*]:
wounds.[282]

{"The country people, the sylvan deities, fauns and his brother satyrs, and Olympus, whom even then he [i.e. Amyas] still loved, the nymphs, all wept for him, and every shepherd who fed his wooly sheep or horned kine on those mountains."}

Ov: met: lb:6. V:392.[283]

when the action was over we encamped near to the field of battle. had violent raine for Sixteen hours, & few tents pitched, many having lost their tent poles, tent pins &c: & no straw. were obliged to lye on wet ground. many men were wet to the skine especially such as were on duty. we had no provision; some men had not broke bread these eight & forty hours[a.]. the wounded were left in the field that night, excepting a few taken up by the enemy. We were like the Roman army commanded by Fabius in Campania, when defeated by the Samnites. viz: in the most unhappy & deplorable condition imaginable, without provisions for the troops, remedies for the sick & wounded, or any means of Reposing themselves, of which they were in so much want [....] the night passed amidst the Groans of the dying, & the complaints of those who survived them. Rollin's Rom:[284]

Men & horses were greatly fatigued & could bear it no longer.

{"Nor could I [i.e., Alcmena] longer bear my pangs. Nay, even now as I tell it, cold horror holds my limbs and my pains return even as I think of it."}

Ov: met: lb:9. V:290.[285]

---

280 Charles Aleyn, *The Battailes of Crescey and Poictiers: under the Fortunes and Valour of King Edward the Third of that Name, and His Sonne Edward Prince of Wales, Named the Black* 2nd ed., enl. (London: Thomas Knight, 1633), p. 50.

281 Hippocrates, Fractures, c.26.

282 Ranby discusses Cumberland's case at length, though referring to the patient (p. 45) only as "a young prince, no less distinguished for his martial prowess, than high birth": *The Method of Treating Gunshot Wounds*, 2nd ed. (London: Robert Horsfield, 1760), pp. 45–5.

283 Ovid, Metamorphoses, 6.392–5.

284 Rollin, *Roman History*, III, 276; "in the ... survived them" is quoted. The reference is to Fabius Gurges, son of Fabius Rullianus Maximus.

285 Ovid, Metamorphoses, 9.289–91.

None of our officers were wounded. Cornet Davis[286] was thrown from his horse, much bruised, being draged & trampled, <vomiting blood,> urine bloody &c:[a.] was

272.

[a.] **{"… angry with himself and his foe alike, and fiercely showing hungry teeth …"}**

Hor. Ep:ii. lib:ii. V.28.[287]

{"You are weak and your veins will fail you, unless food and strong support be given to your sinking stomach."}

Hor: Sat:iii. lib:ii. V:53.[288]

[a.] **{"The red blood spouted forth as he [i.e. Eurytus] lay dying on his back, beating the floor with his head."}**

Ov: met: lb:5. V.83.[289]

273. [*continuing from p. 271*]:
blooded, &c: went to Aix la chapelle for the benefit of the warm bath and recovered dayly. We had many wounded at Fountenoye & such variety of cases that it's impossible to narrate them.

{"'Tis hard to tell of your martial deeds there, how many you gave to death, who they were and how they fell."}

Ov: De Ponto. lb:4. V:335.[290]

there were many contusions from <u>spent Balls</u>, at first sight are small but soon spread, growing black & blew, should be fomented, poulticed, scarified &c: fomentations of herbs smell too strong in a tent; I therefore use milk & water adding some Brandy[a.]. Drought is the most universal complaint from all the wounded, & surgeons would do better in filling their Chests with proper liquors for this purpose, than stuffing them with Apothecaries Drugs; Shrub & water answer this intention. during the cure the body is to kept open by proper dyet.

{"In [a patient] with a fever or a wound, dried bowels is a bad sign."} Hip: de morb:[291]

---

286 John Davis, or Davies, entered the Blues as a cornet on 11 Dec. 1739. He was promoted to lieut. 25 Dec. 1744, but left the regiment, and the army, about July 1745. As Buchanan notes, Davis was the only officer in the Blues who was reported wounded at Dettingen. RADCP 3/47; WO 63/10, f. 8; *The Court and City Register, Compleat for the Year 1744* (London, 1744), p. 10.

287 Horace, Epistles, 2.2.28–9.

288 Horace, Satires, 2.3.153–4.

289 Ovid, Metamorphoses, 5.83–4.

290 Ovid, ex Ponto, 4.7.45–6.

291 Hippocrates, Diseases, 1.7.

our Cuirasses saved many lives <at Fontenoy>, during the action both body & mind are violently agitated, & require some time to settle; here rest is to be indulged, & large bleedings are necessary. many are deeply concerned for the loss of the day [--]

{**"To think so black a sun as this has shone for me!"**}
Hor: Sat:9. lib:1. V:72.[292]

[--] are morose & melancholy, require cheerfull company & a Glass

274.

contusions from cannon balls seldom recover, tho at first they appear to be trieffling, yet soon spread upwards & downwards, commonly attended with large <u>Emphysema</u> over the whole body, as happened to Campbell of Cptn Gilbert's from a bruise on the outside of the right knee; face & body greatly swelled, his very eyes were shut up. & this was the case with many.

{**"All contused wounds, e.g. from fire-arms, were very difficult to cure however slight they were, especially when they were in the head, and and though they were treated with the utmost care they were very often fatal, which brought great discredit on the surgeons; I mean that inflammation would intervene and later gangrene, so that sometimes they were led to suspect that the besieged enemy had poisoned their lead bullets."**}
Ramaz: de morb: artif. cap.42.[293]

Gunshot wounds should be keep'd open a long time, in order to give passage to extranaeous bodies, & when seemingly healed often breake out again from part of the cloaths being forced in with the bullet & not extracted.

{**"Perhaps in long time a scar will form; a raw wound quivers at the touch of a hand. 'Tis not always in a physician's power to cure the sick: at times the disease is stronger than trained art."**}
Ov: de Pont: lib:1. V:247.[294]

275. [*continuing from p. 273*]:
of wine, or to be employed in some new enterprize. Cort: Peruvian: was much used, especially where the Suppuration was large & attended with fever[a].

{**"Those who are wounded should be kept hungry, and their bellies should be cleaned downwards through use of an enema**

---

292 Horace, Satires, 1.9.73.

293 Ramazzini, *De morbis artificum* (trans. Wright), p. 369.

294 Ovid, ex Ponto, 1.3.15–18.

or a purgative. Water or vinegar may be provided."} Hip: de Affect:[295]

Gunshot wounds from being small at first grow dayly larger from a large suppuration of the bruised parts, and are tedious of curing.

{**"Some wounds are made worse by treatment, as we see."**}

Ov: de Pont: lb:3. V:641.[296]

[*margin:* a remarkable Gunshot wound] they are not only confined to the day of battle; are frequent from accidental Shots. Prichard of Cpt. Marcham's was shot by a Dutch Soldier in the Streets of Brussels the ball entering about the middle of the Penis, took off one testicle & bruised the other so much as to render it useless, entered the inner side of the right thigh, passed thro & made it's exit near the Anus. There was no great haemorrhagie: the testicles were taken out as in Castration; the penis cut off about an inch from its root, stiching a small artery. dressed dry covering with digestive, blooded, clystered, drinking Tamarind Ptisane, the parts constantly fomented. there was soon a good digestion. the wound healed surprizingly well from this simple method & was thought a remarkable cure. was naturally healthie & thin habite

276.

[a.] {**Take ½ oz. of *Theriac Andromachi*, 2 oz. powdered Peruvian bark, and *Syrupus caryophillorum*, as required, to make an electuary. A nutmeg-sized dose to be taken every 3 hours.**}

277. [*continuing from p. 275*]:

of body, bearing this misfortune with great patience. his beard never grew afterwards, only a few hairs on the upper lip & round the point of his chin, but not near so strong as formerly; his cheeks are perfectly smooth. nixt Summer did Duty in the field tho not near so strong & heartie as formerly, used to say he was not <u>half the man</u> & never had the least inclination to Venery. he grew dayly more effeminate & of a peevish temper, would cry like a child on the smallest affront, & could not bear the least joacke from any of his comrades, was so troublesome in making frivolous complaints that it was necessary to discharge him[x].

after the action we had many swelled knees, inflammed & painfull from being squeezed in the ranks during the action, & swelled legs were common from so much duty a horseback.

[*margin:* Gunshot wound in horses.] The wounded horses would not foresake their Regmts though they had lost their Riders, & followed so long as they could walk, & some had only three legs to stand on.

he paweth in the valley, & rejoiceth in his Strenght [*sic*], nei-

[295] Hippocrates, Affections, c.38.

[296] Ovid, ex Ponto, 3.7.25–6.

ther turneth he back from the sword, &c: Job: cap: 39.[297] Vid: Buch: Eleg: ad Briand. Vallium[298] et de Equo Elogium.[299]

{**"Behind, the war-steed Aethon, his trappings laid aside, goes weeping, and big drops wet his face."**}
Virg: Aen: xi: V:89.[300]
our Farriers were strangers to Gunshot wounds & I treated some wounded horses much in the same manner as I did the men,

278.
ˣhe afterwards enlisted into General Honeywood's Dragoons & was soon discharged for the same reason. was afterwards in Montague's & turn'd out for the same reason.
{**"For war are horses armed, war these herds portend."**}
Virg: Aen: 3–540.[301]

279. [*continuing on from p. 277*]
Viz: extracting the bullet, digesting &c.

The wounded are often neglected as to dayly dressings, especially after a general action, Corpll. Orford of Sr James's was not dressed for ten days after I amputated his forearm, tho he was sent from camp to the Hospital. the part stunke abominably, the dressings were almost rotted, a large discharge of sharp stinking matter, & a long bare stump; but did well with proper care. he often imagined he wanted to stir the fingers of that hand, & in the night time would often start as if something pricked them. it's the same with toes after the amputation of the leg, they even complaine of their corns aching. the Corpll fainted at the beginning of

297 v. 21–2.

298 Buchanan apparently has in mind these lines from George Buchanan's elegy, "*Ad Briandum Vallium, Senatorem Burdegal, pro Lena apologia*" ("To Briand de Vallee, Public Official of Bordeaux, an apology for the Procuress"): "For though the spirited horse may be broken by inactive old age, when the harsh horns have given the war signals, he rages in his mind, he strikes the earth with his hoof, he pricks up his ears, still retaining his fighting spirit though his powers are failing"; Sabrio, "Buchanan's *Elegies*," p. 63.

299 Buchanan's Silva VI, "*De equo elogium*" ("A Short Statement concerning the Horse"), includes the passage, "If battles call, keen energy flows into its trembling joints, and with its master it pours forth a shared rage from the mouth and nostrils. And it exposes its noble breast to wounds, and alone with its master, it takes and lays aside the joys and sorrows in every chance": ibid., p. 158.

300 Virgil, Aeneid, 11.89–90.

301 Ibid., 3.540.

the operation & did not know he had lost his arm till he obsserv'd the dressings*

[*margin:* Deseases after the Battle.] The day after the battle of Dettenghem we encamped twixt Hanau & Francfort on the Banks of the Mayne, & were well supplyed with all sorts of provision <but no straw the first night>.

[*margin:* Grieps & purging.] Many men complained of grieps & purging, saying, they got cold the night of the battle;

[*margin:* Method of cure.] as they have frequent reachings to vomite I order a Dose of Ipecacuan: & op: h:S: & a Dose Rhabarb with Nutmeg nixt morning, repeating the opiate, & continuing this method three or four days, compleating the cure with Discord dr.i in burnt Gin every night at bedtime. this was the most common distemper in our hospital & treated such in the same manner. if this Desease continued some time the Stools

280.

***{"They tell how scythed chariots, reeking with indiscriminate slaughter, often shear off a limb so suddenly, that it is seen to quiver on the ground when it falls shorn from the trunk, although the man's mind and strength from the swiftness of the blow can feel no pain; and at the same time, because the mind has been absorbed in the ardour of battle, with what is left of his body, he pursues battle and blood."}**

Lucret. de rerum natura. lib:iii. V.643.[302]

281. [*continuing from p. 279*]:
grew bloody, attended with all the complaints of the Bloody-Flux. I then ordered {**six gr. *Vitrum ceratum antimonii* and ½ gr. *Theriac Andromachi* to make a pill to be taken in the morning. An opium pill should be taken at bedtime.**} this being continued some days many recovered in Camp tho reduced to great weaknes[a]. this encreased so much by the midle of July that five or Six of a troop were ill at one time; the weather being dry favoured their recovery. by the midle of Augst it was so common that I could not keep a list of the mens names or cases; the Vitr: cerat: Antim: was the universal medicine & never failed to stop the bleeding, excepting two cases, & Diascord in Burnt Gin seldom failed of removing the grieps. the Grieps were always in the lower belly, twixt the Navel & os Pubis, the sick man commonly covering the part with his hand as he told his complaints[b]. as the complaints were in the lower belly there was no occasion for vomits; there was seldom any fever & bleeding was never used in Camp; but in the Hospital many recovering, fevered & dye.

---

[302] Lucretius, de Rerum Natura, 3.642–8.

[*margin:* our hospital in great disorder.] Here our hospital was in great disorder as their baggage was not yet arrived from Flanders, the Sick lyeing on straw only in Barns, Stables, outhouses, &c: there was commonly a Dunghill befor the Door where all their Pots, Bedpans, &c: were emptied, & stinke abominably in warm weather, & great swarms of vermine are dayly produced*; those Dunghills are lower situated than the Street, & when raine falls the common Channel empties

282.

[a.] our Allies knew nothing of this medecine, so treated it with small Doses Ipecacaon: & Rhabarb. & some of our Surgeons do the same, never making tryale of Vitr. Cerat: Antimon: & probably the good success from it may be in a great measure owing to my persisting in its use.

[b.] when the tenesmus is troublesome I have used clysters of burnt Claret with Theria: Androm: & that with good success. especially where the parts are weakened by the long continuance of the Desease, & the patient complaining when he stands upright, that he perceives his bowells, as it were, bearing downwards. they are seldom used amongst the men, having a foolish aversion to them. vid Young on Opium Sect. 8th[,] the effects of Opium in the Tenesmus.[303] vid Fred: Hoffman: Op: Med: Tom:3. p. 151. de Dysenteria.[304]

*Fred: Hoffmanni Op: Med: Tom:i. p.207. de Venenis in Aere contentis Epidemionum Morborum Causis.[305]

283. [*continuing on from p. 281*]:
itself into the Dunghills, carrying much filth along with it, & after raine the stench was almost insufferable[a.]. vid: Degneri hist: medic: de Dysenteria.[306]

> **{"However, of all the causes that introduce these legions of diseases into a camp, not one does as much harm in my opinion as the filth and neglect of personal cleanliness in the camp itself. The Israelites of old were forbidden by a divine statute to**

---

[303] Young, *Treatise on Opium*, sect. 8, esp. pp. 53–5. Young asserts that opium can be helpful in treating tenesmus, but that if the stimulus is too great it cannot contain it.

[304] *Opera omnia*, part III (vol. III), sect. ii, ch. 7, pp. 156, 157; cf. *System of the Practice of Medicine*, II, 179, 183. Opiates play a very small part in the treatment outlined by Hoffmann.

[305] "*De venenis in aere contentis epidemiorum morborum causis*" ("Of airborne poisons that cause epidemic diseases"); Hoffmann, *Opera omnia*, I, pars ii, cap. v, pp. 207–12. Hoffmann asserts that airborne matter or creatures that may cause disease and epidemics.

[306] Johann Hartmann Degner [Degneri], *Historia medica de dysenteria bilioso-contagiosa* (Utrecht, 1738); Degner discusses the role of filth in spreading dysentery on pp. 53–4.

venture to void faeces within the camp; it must be done outside the camp .... This is the passage in Deuteronomy [chapter 23; *Buchanan's interpolation*]: 'Thou shalt have a place without the camp whither thou shalt go for the calls of nature; and thou shalt have a paddle with thy weapons, and when thou hast eased thyself thou shalt turn back and cover that which cometh from thee; for thy God walketh in the midst of thy camp.'"}
Ramaz: de morb: Artif. Cap:42.[307]

[*margin:* flux & fevers are universal & very mortal.] fevers & fluxes were almost universal, & thought infectious; few Apothecaries or their Mates escaping one or other of those deseases, & many dyed; the Nurses dyed so fast that private Soldiers were obliged to nurse their Comrades. We suffered more from this sickness than from the day of battle. it put me in mind of the plague in the Roman & Carthaginian Army at the Siege of Syracuse. Viz: 'at first the distemper was moderate, & occasioned only by the bad air & Season, afterwards communication with the Sicke, & even the care taken of them, spread the contagion: from whence it happened that some, neglected and abandoned, dyed thro the malignity of the Desease, others received help that became fatale to all that approached them, so that the eyes were continually strucke with the sad sight of death, & of the funerals that followed it, & the ears

284. [a] {**"There is no house here well suited to a sick man, no beneficial food for him, none to relieve, with Apollo's art, his pain, no friend to comfort, none to beguile with talk the slow-moving hours. Aweary I lie among these far-away peoples in this far-away place, and thoughts come to me in my weakness of everything that is not here."**}
Ov: trist: lib:iii. V:121.[308]

[*margin:* French Hospital.] the day after the battle I was sent to the French camp in order to visite the wounded of our Army. their Surgeons went round the hospital carrying a tub of Brandy & Syringes, with which they washed the wounds, dressing with dry lint dipt in brandy, & covering with digestive. Such of their wounded as could be transported & require time to recover, were sent to the nearest French towns. the wounded lay on Strawe or hay in houses, churches, Barns &c: our men say the French bleed often & cut much.

[*margin:* Hanoverian hospital.] The Hanoverians had their hospital baggage in the field; their hospital was soon put in good order; their men in good houses, lye on palliases stuffed with Straw, have good coverings; their dressings are very neat of drawn lint, wounds cleaned with fine Spunge, soaked in warm water & brandy, use the caustic on the first

---

[307] Ramazzini *De morbis artificum* (trans. Wright), pp. 359, 361.
[308] Ovid, Tristia, 3.3.9–14.

appearance of proud flesh. their common Digestive is Lint Arcaei with ol: Ovor: their hospital medecines are carried on a large waggon, divided into many different partitions, & opening at many places; any particular medicine may be easely got at, the whole easely packed & unpacked. one of their Physicians visits the kitchene dayly & examines the provision. their Regimental Surgeons charge what medecines they use & are paid by the public; use many chemical preparations & great variety of Specieses &c:

> {**"Medical treatment in camps is not as unskilled and irregular as people think, and ... princes and commanders of armies take care that they and their troops shall have skilful doctors furnished with an ample supply of medicines, and they pay these doctors large salaries. This was so in the Trojan War, for we read that the physician Machaon, a celebrated surgeon, accompanied the Greek army."**}
>
> Ramaz: de morb: Artific: C:42.[309]

[*margin:* Dutch hospital.] The Dutch seldom use praecipitate in dressing wounds thinking it too corrosive; their's is seldom good, being much adulterated with Minium & remains unactive like red lead; mel: Rosar: their chief detergent. tereb: cum vitello ovi solut. their common digestive, fomenting chiefly with red wine. when in garrison often agree with the town hospital to take care of their men & provide dyet & medecine for twelve pence pr day.

285. [*continuing on from p. 283*]:
heard nothing night & day but the groans of the dying & those who lamented them. Roll: Rom: hist:[310]

I attended the hospital dayly, yet never had the least Complaint[c]. when I suspected a beginning mortefication of the Bowells, or observed livid Spots on the skine, I ordered extract: Cort: Peruvian: Bark & often succeeded well. Ryce gruell with cinnamon was their common drink, & Ryce gruell their chief dyet. small milk punch was common drink in Camp. living on mutton broth with Ryce or Barley. Some men eat a pennyworth of Blea Berries <Bill Berries, or Vitis Idea> every morning, & found them of great service in stopping the flux. it was common to all, even to such as did not eat fruite, nor drink beer, nor eat Ammonition bread. Some think it occasioned amongst the men from eating their flesh meat too new killed, but we did so long befor the desease appeared[a]. more probably from the bad provision befor the battle & great fatigue & violent raine thereafter[b].

---

309 Ibid., pp. 361, 363.

310 Rollin, *Roman History*, V, 210–11.

{"Therefore, all diseases arise partly from things inside the body – phlegm and bile – and no doubt partly from things outside it – toil and wounds – as well as from heat that makes it too hot and cold that makes it too cold, dryness that makes it too dry and moisture that makes it too humid."} Hip: de Morb: lib:1[311] et de vict: rat: lb:3.

{"But when, as the body grows hot, the purging becomes harsh, the intestine is scraped and ulcerated, and the stools are bloody; this intestinal trouble is called dysentery, a difficult and dangerous disease."}[312]

Many thought it infectious, of which I have no certain proof. it decreased about

286.

[c] Some constitutions are proof against infection. Socrates, by temperance & constant perseverance in the virtuous toil of martial exercises, acquired a constitution superior to the attacks of Disease; for when an almost universal plague had seized upon the Camp, insomuch that more than Eleven hundred men were carried off by contagion in the army before Potidaea, & Athens itself was half depopulated, he escaped in both places the malady, & was the only one in the first that had not in some measure felt the Severity of it. vid: The life of Socrates, by John Gilbert Cooper, jun: Esqr. Lond. 1749. 8[vo.313]

[a] **{"Too often our poor soldiers survive the risks of fire and sword in some campaign only to be overtaken by a host of maladies; armies are almost always decimated by some malignant epidemic. Camp fevers, then, and other fatal and contagious diseases are famous or rather infamous."}**

Ramaz: de morb: Artif: C:42.[314]

[b] It was not known among the Hessians nor Hanoverians, nor any other troops who were not at the battle, nor were any of the country people seized with it.

{"During incessant, heavy rain, the diseases that generally arise are protracted fevers, fluxes of the bowels, mortifications, epilepsy, apoplexy, and angina, but in dry weather occur consumption, inflammations of the eye, pains in the joints, strangury, and dysentery."}

---

311 Hippocrates, Diseases, I, 1.

312 Hippocrates, Regimen, III, 74.

313 Cooper, *The Life of Socrates: Collected from the Memorabilia of Xenophon and the Dialogues of Plato* (London: R. Dodsley, 1749), p. 25; "by temperance … Severity of it" is quoted.

314 Ramazzini, *De morbis artificum* (trans. Wright), p. 359.

Hip: Aph: No.16. S:iii.[315]

287. [*continuing from p. 285*]:
the end of Augst, only two of the Regmt dyed viz: Qr. Master Barbar,[316] he had it to a violent degree, voiding pure foetid blood with many white philms on his first complaint; never was better of any medecine; of an unwholesome swarthy complexion; thought he got a cold a foraging[a]. Livins of Sr James's was the only private man. had been some time in the hospital & under a mercurial course, upon coming to camp, catched cold, & dyed of this Distemper, nor was he in the least relieved by any medecine.

[*margin:* fruite not to be blamed as the principale cause.] fruite is always blamed as the principale cause of this disorder, especially grapes & Plumbs, yet none were large enough to be gathered when the disorder made its first appearance, & we see it decline when the fruite is in plenty. I have known a Soldier have the Bloody flux to a great degree; who never tasted fruite from a natural aversion. Officers eat much more fruit than private men, yet in our German Campn. only two of our Officers were ill of this Distemper.

[*margin:* Bloody flux in Campn. 1744.] This disease appeared in Campn 1744 about the midle of Augst the weather at that time wet & rainy, & was preceeded all summer by a slight Diarhea. the above method proved successfull, for none of the Regmt dyed. it was peculiar to the Soldier, none of the Officers having the least Dysenterick complaint, & only one Qr. Master. nor were any women or children ill of it. We had fruite in abundance, tho Plumbs were forbid by publicke order. this flux was more obstinate than in Germany, tho the blood Stopt, yet the scouring continued, probably from being so late in the Season, & the best medecine was warm cloathing,

288.
[a] he was said to have almost starved himself by a poor dyet three weeks befor. I recommend a good dyet, warm clothing, & good Wine with cheerfull company as the best preservative.

[b] there was but one Dysenterick in Windsor Camp 1740, viz: Hall of Capt. Gilbert's. yet all sorts of summer fruits were eaten in great plenty, but we had little or no fatigue, nor night grand Guards. the Season dry & warm, plenty of Straw for the mens tents. the Regmt was remarkably healthie; some slight feverish complaints, Pleuretick or Rheumaticke, sore throats. only one man dyed during that Campn. viz: Marriot of the Kings, of the dry belly ach, & thought it proceeded from eating too freely of

---

315 Hippocrates, Aphorisms, III, 16.
316 Untraceable.

Salt Bacon not well boyled; & swallowing many cherry Stones of late. in Campn 1745 Septr 29th there was neither flux nor Ague in the Regmt. tho we had plenty of fruite; there was no hard Duty.

[*margin:* a Lady, subject to hysterick cholicks, but is free from complaints of this kind during the Summer Season & eats freely of fruite, yet Green Tea occasions cholicky complaints, but not so with Bohea.]

This is the most universal Camp desease: it appeared in Wm the Conqueror's Army, with which he was himself seized as he marched towards London after the Battle of Hastings[;] vid Carte's Genll. hist: of Engld Vol.1. lib:5 p.391. fol.[317]

The English army in Ireland commanded by Marshall Schomberg, were encamped near Dundalk, which being <a> marshy, unwholesome place, half his troops soon died of fluxes &c. Parker's memoirs of the military transactions in Ireland, &c: p.16.

289. [*continuing on from p. 288*]:
viz: flannel westcoat nixt the skin & socks on the feet. Diascord was given in burnt brandy, the Gin being not so good as in Germany, & the German Gin seemed more effectuale.

> {**"Whatever herb potent for aid, whatever root that is used for healing grows in all the world, is mine."**}
>
> Ov: Ep: 5. V:47.[318]

such Regmts as came lately from England were more subject to it, than those who stood the Campn last year[a]. We had many private receipts as infallible, but I would rather trust good nursing than family medecines, nor do I think this disorder so dangerous as is commonly reported; people are alarmed at the very name of blood, & when they begin to faint & weake, which is the consequence of all fluxes, they impute <it> to the quantity of blood they have lost, tho it may be, does not amount to a Spoonfull or two. Nor does blood always appear at first, being rather the consequence of violent straining; as violent blowing the nose brings first some drops of blood & then a bleeding. it generally appears first amongst the foot; they have harder Duty than the horse & not so well cloathed.

[*margin:* The men have their own particular method of cure.]
Many men attempt curing themselves, by eating hard boyled eggs, old cheese toasted, boyled milk thickened with eggs, abstaining from liquids of all kinds, &c: but soon grow sicke at Stomach, complaining of weight & loade, retching to vomite, but bring up nothing. & I have often been obliged to give two or more vomits in order to remove these complaints. I have used Ipecacoan: gr.vi. in a Glass of wine every fourth hour with

---

[317] Thomas Carte, *A General History of England* (London: printed for the author, 1747), I, bk. v, p. 391.

[318] Ovid, Heroides, 5.147–8.

good success. it occasioned frequent retchings but seldom vomited. In England the inner pyth of Walnuts viz

290.

[a]Chomley's Regt. had upwards of thirty men ill, about the beginning of Septr.

291. [*continuing on from p. 289*]:
that which divides the Kernel into four parts, is esteemed as infallible in this diorder [*sic*], if taken in powder or steep'd in Brandy & taken by way of Dram. Mr. Douglas, Surgn to the Welch-Fuziliers,[319] gave it to some of his men, without any more effect than a Dram of plaine Brandy. to the taste it's gently astringent[a].

[*margin:* Bloody flux in Campn 1745.] This Desease appeared in Campn. 1745, about the midle of May, from catching cold during the preceeding wet weather, & fatigue at the battle of Fountenoye. it was not universal, being confined to such troops only, as had most fatigue. alarms were so frequent amongst our out parties, that there was scarce time to pitch tents, or untye cloaks, all lay on the cold ground exposed to the open air, & tho the days were warm the nights were cold. they were not very obstinate; the dry weather afterwards favoured their cure. the month of June was more like winter than Summer & many relapsed, the weather was so wet & cold that medecines could not be given in Camp. all Dysentericks were sent to the Hospital, & if they returned to camp befor their health was well established, they were sure to relapse & be useless that Season. Now fruite is not blamed, there being at this Season no such thing;yet irregularity must be charged to the poor Soldier & gin is blamed; yet I have always observed the drunken Soldier the most healthie, but when seized with Sickness, often attended with greatest danger. the weather was dry & warm next Septr. & we had no such disorder, tho we had fruite in great plenty but no

292. [a]the yolke of an egg beaten with a lump of fine Sugar, adding a Glas brandy is recommended as an infallible remedy. I often advise it to our men on their recovery, as a nourishing cordial, taken in the morning befor we march.

---

[319] James Douglas was commissioned surgeon to the Fusiliers (23rd Foot) 19 April 1742 and held the post until 19 June 1752. In August 1750 he received his M.D. from Aberdeen (Mariscal.); according to Anderson, he was "Present himself and examined and came off with great applause." He may have been the James Douglas MCS who as of 1783 was practicing at Bedford Square. *Medical Register for 1783*, p. 19; Anderson, *Fasti Academiae Mariscallanae Aberdonensis*, p. 116; Johnston's *Roll*, pp. 11 (#195), 13 (#238 [note: Johnston incorrectly identifies him with another James Douglas]).

293. [*continuing from p. 291*]:
great fatigue from Camp: Duty. this desease has never been attended with that dangerous fever as in the hospital in Germany. I always imagined that fever proceeded chiefly from the bad air & stinking vapour of that nasty place. here is the same Disorder tho not so frequent, a neat clean hospital, well aired, & not much crowded. which was just the reverse in Germany & that in a violent hot Summer. Some Dysentericks had hard swelled bellies, & were more common with the foot than horse; were difficult of cure; Saponaceous & mercurial medecines were prescribed, poultices, &c: issues cut in the thighs, few recovered, many dyeing Dropsical. this was not know<n> amongst our men <Troopers>.

[*margins:* Dysentericks dissected.] Such Dysenterics as were desected, their intestines from the Colon were mortified & remarkably so near the Anus; the bladder ready to mortifie & so tender that it was easely tore to pieces, tho gently handled. the Stomach in tollerable good order. the body had a strong putride smell, & the Dissector often imagined himself indisposed nixt day, being sicke at Stomach & grumbling pains in his bowells; fearing infection took a Vomite & Dose Rhubarb.

[*margin:* Camp fever 1743.] a Slowe fever appeared about the end of Augst in Campn 1743. attended with violent headach, watchfulnes, faintness & universal weakness. pulse so low that bleeding did not seem proper, a constant drought.

[*margin:* Method of Cure.] all drunk freely of Rhenish wine & water & found great benefite from the Op: pill: when given in large quantities. viz: {up to ½ gr. of purified opium.} blisters behind the ears were of great service. Decoct: Serpentar: the chief medecine & Camphorated boluses. those who recovered

294. [*facing p. 293; blank*]

295. [*continuing from p. 293*]
continued faint and weak many days, greatly low-Spirited, & despairing of doing well, & fearing being left behind. which is always the case with Soldiers & greatly prevents recovery, their Mind being never easie[a]. I ordered Assafoetid: scr.i. pr diem with a Glas strong wine, & proved a good medecine, & so was the Barke infused with wine. this was very common & greatly resembling the Lingring fever in Par: 10th. Rushworth of Sir James's dyed Sept. 22d. in the hospital: all sorts of medecines were tryed but to no purpose, nor had they any visible effect. his looks were always naturale but his voice sunke & broke. would eat & drink such things as were offered but never called for any. Munke of Capt. Shipman's dyed the Sixth day, would neither eat nor drink, nor taste medecines, saying he was certaine he must dye, & did dye in his tent. our men had taken a dislike to the hospital, would rather suffer the injuries of the

weather in the field, or think themselves happy if they got into a Boners out-house & lye on straw. Many nurses & children dyed & it seemed to be more mortal with them than with the men.

[*margin:* Bleeding is prejudicial in some fevers[x].] About the midle of Septr. I had twelve men ill of this fever & all lay in houses adjoining our camp, one insisted on being blooded, which I did in order to please him; he was more faint & weake than formerly, & longer a recovering than any of his Comrades. the Officers enquiring after their Sicke men & hearing they had fevers, naturally asked if they had been blooded, & upon answering in the negative, they seemed angry as if I had neglected them[.]

> **{"either because they think nothing can be right, save what has pleased themselves ..."}**[a].
>
> Hor: Ep:1. lb:2. V:83.[320]

they imagined bleeding was necessary in all fevers. this <was> often attended

296.

[a] when delirious in fevers talk of their horses, arms, accoutrements, &c: & Rollin in vol: 10th Roman: Hist: observes of Marius that he abandoned himself to excesses of the table, & passed his nights in drinking with his friends. by this regimen he soon inflammed his blood. he was taken with a fever, which presently seized his head, & in his delirium he raved on nothing but the war with Mithridates. he imagined that he had the command of it, & not when he spoke, but made gestures & assumed the attitudes of a man that fights, or of a General giving orders. so violent & incurable was the passion & so deeply had it taken over in his heart, with which ambition & jealousy uniting, had inspired him for that command.[321] and our men after the battle of Fontenoye raved of entrenchments, batteries, Dispositions &c

> [x] **{"[We observed in the Xenodochium] That in acute Diseases, most of those whose Blood drawn by Venesection had a white chylous Crust upon it, recover'd; and those dy'd, whose Blood was very rutilant, or had too red a Surface."}**
>
> Bagl. Prax: Med: lib:1. C.13.[322]

Tissot on Bilious fevers, does not approve of bleeding[.] p.180.[323]

> [a] **{"What would you have me do? After all, men have not all the same tastes and likes."}**

---

320 Horace, Epistles, 2.1.83.

321 Rollin, *Roman History*, X, 46; "abandon[ed] himself ... that command" is quoted.

322 Baglivi, *The Practice of Physick*, p. 166; *De praxi medica*, I, cap. xiii, p. 120. There is a possibility that Buchanan took this passage not directly from Baglivi, but rather from Johnstone, who also quotes it (*Historical Dissertation*, p. 56).

323 Tissot, *Essay on Bilious Fevers*, pp. 179–85.

Hor: Ep:ii: lib:ii V:57.[324]

297. [*continuing on from p. 295*]:
with inflammation of the eyes. Lieut. Pawlet[325] dyed the 23d. day at Worms. was treated in the same manner as Rushworth, nor had medecines any better effect. was remarkably healthie & hardy, never made use of a bedstead, always laying on Straw on the ground, & says he got cold. Qr. Mr. Cumbers[326] dyed in the hospital after a month's illnes exactly in the same <manner> as the Lieut & <it> was remarkable that he & Qr. Mr. Barbar always lay on Straw upon <the ground>, & these three were the <only> Officers who dyed in this Campn. this fever continued to the end of the Campn. <& was always a constant attendant on the Army.> all complained of catching cold. as this was our first campn the men might be more easely affected. 'it is observed in Authors, that the Roman Army which made war in so many climates, perish seldom much with sickness, whereas it often happens now a days, that armies without engaging, lie dead on the field. Roll: in his preface to the Rom: Hist:[327] but their Youth were more accustomed to labour & hardships, & we were just come from good quarters & strangers to the Camp life[a].

> {**[Of the early Romans:] "To begin with, as soon as the young men could endure the hardships of war, they were taught a soldier's duties in camp under a vigourous discipline, and they took more pleasure in handsome arms and war horses than in harlots and revelry. To such men consequently no labour was unfamiliar, no region too rough or too steep, no armed foeman was terrible; valour was all in all. Nay, their hardest struggle for glory was with one another; each man strove to be first to strike down the foe, to scale a wall, to be seen of all while doing such a deed. This they considered riches, this fair fame and high nobility."**} Sall: in bell: Catilini.[328]
>
> {**"In the days of old this was the training and the delight of youth, these were the skills which formed the leaders of the future –**

298.

many thought this was a new distemper, the like being never known, but men read in Biograph. Britann. Art. Spelman. he was seized with the

---

[324] Hor. Ep. 2.2.57–8; *Horace* (trans. Fairclough), p. 429.

[325] John Pawlet had entered the Blues as a cornet 2 Oct.1731 and had been promoted to lieut., 10 Dec. 1739. WO 64/10, f. 8; *AL 1740*, p. 6.

[326] Untraceable.

[327] Rollin, *Roman History*, I, xxiii–xxiv; "observed ... field" is quoted.

[328] Sallust, Cataline, 7.4–6.

camp-desease at Brazen Nose College, which put an end to his life July 25th 1644.[329]

[a.] at the Siege of Agrigentum they were greatly distressed both by famine, & deseases which are always the effect of it. & at the Seige of Lilybaeum they were forced to subsist chiefly on horse flesh, & 10,000 dyed in a short time. Roll: Rom: hist.[330] & Pompey ruined his army by continuing the Siege of Numantia during the winter, the rigor of the Season, & the air & water of the country, to which those Soldiers were not accustomed, occasioned many diseases, & particularly very painfull cholicks, which made a great havocke in the Army. Roll: Rom: hist: vol. 8th.[331] see Reflections on the Causes of the Rise & fall of the Roman Empire, by M: de Secondat. Lond. 1752. 8$^{vo.}$ Chap. 2d. of the Science of war as practised by the Romans.[332]

[*interleaved between pp. 297 and 298 (glued to p. 297)*]

N.B: a fever of this nature appeared at Stone in Staffordshire 1752. & was brought there by the Welch Fuzileers in marching from N: to S: some of their Sick were left here & continued in a lingring [*word obliterated*] condition for sometime; the poor family where they were quartered soon sickened & were a long time afflicted with a slowe-lingring fever, their nixt neighbour catched it, & it soon becam general amongst the poor people nor did the better sort [*crossed out:* of people] escape it, nor was it confined to the town only, for it soon got into the Neighbouring Farmhouses, & at the time is very frequent & mortal – vid Regimental Practice M.S: p. 297. (March 29th 1753)

[*crossed out:* it Returned in Aprl 1753]

Nov. 1755. it appeared at Stafford among the Poor-people & many dyed without help. last Summer it was in the neighbouring villages, & it was remarkable that four people dyed in one house. Dr. James's powder has been tryed sometimes in full Doses, & sometimes ½. promotes Stools & slight reachings, but seldom Sudorific. unless from Regm. its much in Eccleshall workhouse

April 1756. it continues at Stafford, chiefly confined to poor people & Prisoners, workhouses. the Jailors wife dyed; James's powder was the chief medecine, had no visible effect May 6th. the jaile's Situation low &

329 *Biog. Brit.*, VI, pt. i, p. 3793; "he was seized … 1644" is quoted. The entry on Sir John Spelman does not provide any other details on the nature or course of the disease. Spelman actually died in 1643.

330 Rollin, *Roman History*, IV, 39, 103; "were greatly … effect of it" and "to subsist … short time" are quoted.

331 Ibid., VIII, 253–4; "during the … the army" is quoted.

332 Charles Louis de Secondat, baron de Montesquieu, *Reflections on the Causes of the Rise and Fall of the Roman Empire*, 2nd ed., enl. (London: W. Innys [etc.], 1752).

damp. The justices at the last meeting ordered the feverish Prisoners to be removed from the Dungeon to an upper room to have a bed & firing &c. winter wet & open[.] One woman recovered without any medecine; small whey or Chamomel Tea was her only drink, & a blister was applied when very low. viz: Mrs. Hordine.

April 1758. many are sick in Jaile, the Justices ordered three hundered wt. of Coals pr. week, & double quantity of Straw; the judge recommended Ventilators, & the Sheriff to have an open Casement in each window &c.

[*interleaved between pp. 297 and 298; loose; apparently a later draft of preceding*]

N:B: a fever of this nature appeared at Stone in Staffordshire Feby 1752. & was brought there by the Welch Fuziliers in marching from N: to S: some of their sicke were left [*crossed:* here] and continued in a lingring condition [*crossed:* for] sometime; the poor family where they were quartered soon sickened & were a long while afflicted with a slowe lingring fever, their nixt neighbour catched it, & it soon became general among the poor people, & many dyed without any help. nor was it confined to the town only, for it soon got into the neighbouring farm houses, nor did the better sort escape it, & is at this time is very frequent & mortal.

Novr. 1755. it appeared at Stafford among the poor people & many dyed; last Summer it was in the neighbouring villages, & it was remarkable that four people died in one house. it is much in Eccleshall workhouse.

April 1756. it continued at Stafford but chiefly confined to poor people & Prisoners, the Jailors wife died, & some Prisoners. the Jail's Situation lowe & damp, winter wet & cold, so many Prisoners sicke that the Apory was afraid to attend them. The Justices at their last meeting were so humane to the unhappy Prisoners as to order the sicke in the Dungeon to be removed to an upper room to be allowed a Bed & firing for which the County made an allowance of I sh. pr. weeke, & many recovered without much medecine. <the dirty Straw to be burnt, & a greater quantity of fresh allowed weekly.> a poor woman took only small whey & Chamomile tea for some weeks, with the help of a Blister did well.

Aprl 1758 Many Prisoners were sicke & could not take their tryale at the Spring Ass[izes] & the Judges were cautious, for fear of infection. <3 poor folks dyed in one house in the forehead.> The Justices at last Sessions granted further indulges to the Prisoners by allowing them three hundered weight of Coals weekly from the first of Octr. to the 1st. of May, & double quantity of Straw. Ventilators have been recommended <& put up>, or having an open Casement in each roome. our Summer

Assizes are nixt week, & there is not one feverish Prisoner, nor do I know of any in town. this fever has raged greatly at Congleton some years, appeared at first among the working folks at the Silk Mill; some imagined the infection was brought home with the Silk. it was very mortal, Apothecaries, Surgeons, Nurses &c: dyed. & some of the principal inhabitants. some families left the place for fear of infection. it was common among the Potters at Henley Green, Boslem & Stoke, especially with the poorer sort, nor did the better sort escape it. Mr. Keeline of Henley Green died July 20th, after two weeks illness.

Spring 1758. it appeared at Leeke amongst the workers of Moyhair & Silk & was confined to them only, was thought to be imported with those commodities. it encreased towards Summer, in Augst. Mr. Jackson one of the chief Manufacturers lost two sons in one week, & had twenty seven workmen ill of this fever; & another Workman had Sixteen of his Servants down of it at the same time. they generally dye about the Eleventh day. have <many> red, black & blew Spots on their skins; such as come to suppuration have a chance to recover.

Winter 1759. it was much at Eccleshall[.] Young Mr. Garrison laboured under it upwards of Six weeks & recovered to the surprize of all his neighbours. it was thought infectious as others of the family were seized with it as also some of his Nurses; it run through the Apothecaries family[.]

Summer 1760 it appeared in Mrs. Dickinson's boarding School at Stafford. few of the children escaped it. it was said to be occasioned from eating fruite, of which there is great plenty, especially pears. sickness at Stomach their first complaint with reaching to vomite & soon after loose stools, frothy & foetid. Ementicks & cathartics were always used & at first were successfull & often put an end to all complaints. some laboured under it many days, were treated with mild acescent drinks, Rhubarb in small Doses, gentle cordials[.]

about the latter end of Octr 1761 it was very common at Stafford & only among the poor people & such as live near the River & damp places, viz: the broad eye, & Mill-Lane, the Green &c: whole families are down, three in a bed, are miserably poor, having scarcely the common necessaries of life, no fire. Emeticks with Camamile tea [&] vinegar whey are the universal medecines. infusions of snakeroot, to a poor <woman> it was given by way of Clyster with immedeate good effect. many die. last Summer was remarkably dry & warm & so was the harvest, but suddenly changed to wet & cold. its common in the workers. at Newport, where many die. at Stafford the better sort of people generously collected in order to support the poor with good nursing wch proved the best medecine. towards Xmas it decreased as the weather became dry & frosty. Dr. James's powder was only given to one poor woman & she died.

299. [*continuing from p. 297*]:

> **to pit speed against an animal's swift-footedness, and strength and dexterity against its courage and; while in times of peace it brought no small honour to sweep marauding beasts from the plains and raise the siege they laid to the farmers and their work."**} Plin:[333]

Many men relapsed on their return to camp, & being put too soon on Duty; when I order them to Camp I give a certificate excusing a week's Duty, especially from night Guards or out-parties.

> {**"If, owing to violent exertion, [the patient] becomes emaciated, let him give it up, relax, and rest. When he has recovered, he should not run speedily into the wind, nor mount a horse or a chariot, and he should avoid shouting and excitement; for there is a danger that the disease will return .... For if you do not take care of him after he has been restored to health, unless he takes care of himself, the disease often returns, causing death .... If he exerts himself by riding in a chariot or on a horse, or exhausts himself by placing a burden on his shoulders, he faces a danger that the disease will come back, and if this happens there is a danger that he will be destroyed. The disease, on returning, presses harder than it did at the beginning .... Above all, keep him quiet, and give him suitable food."**} Hip: de intern: affect:[334]

[*margin:* Rheumatism.] By the latter end of Septr* 1743. Rheumatick Stiches with pain <in> bones were common, the limbs benumbed that they could scarcely move them in the morning, from catching cold in the night time. tho the days were dry & pleasant, yet the nights were cold & frosty air, winds often easterly. & used to have ten or twelve complaining every morning, the pulse quick & full, required bleeding. Bol: ad Rheumatismum Nostr. with Op: was the chief medecine. it was needless to attempt sweating in tents at this Season. were sent to the neighbouring villages, had warm roomes with Stoves, were sweated with Success; the knees were often swelled

---

333 Pliny, Panegyricus, 81.2.

334 Hippocrates, Internal Affections, 1.8.

300.
*vid: Hoffman: Op: Med: Tom:3. p:63. de temporibus Anni Insalubribus.[335] & p.70 de Siderum in Corpora humana, influxu Medico.[336]

301. [*continuing on from p. 299*]:
and stiff; much swelled, red & painfull; fomentations of great Service, rubbing with Ungt. Vol: nost: & covering with flannel.

{**"Whenever pain is present, warm baths and fomentations help to soften whichever part of the leg pain happens to settle in, and to evacuate the bowels. And when the pain is washed away, give a medication to purge downwards."**} Hip: de affect:[337]

{**"From this disease many become lame."**} Ib: de intern: affect:[338]

{**"[The patient] should observe as light a diet as possible .... But the disease is difficult and prolonged."**} Ib.[339]

Lafters of Cptn Gilberts was thirty days in the hospital for an obstinate Rheumatism, never the better of any medecines unless he sweated; was sweated one and twenty nights successively & recovered, but continued weake sometime. Sap: castiliens: pulveris: is used by some as a favorite medecine in this case; is powdered by toasting before a gentle fire in a paper bag, & given ab dr.fs. ad dr.i. in milk, whey or small beer. Is much commended in the Gravale & jaundice. I have often seen the good effects of a whey dyet in Rheumaticks, but it's impossible to perswade a Soldier to continue it a sufficient time. Opiates were of the greatest service, especially when given in large Doses, ad gr.ii. op: pur: with something warm, a good night's rest was always procured & sweats promoted, & seldom or never observed any bad effects from this free use of Opium, but am convinced it's the most universal medecine for soldiers. it became a universal practice, & the pure Opium is equal to any of it's preparations. should be kept moiste or beat up with Sap. otherwise it grows dry & hard, passing thro the body without any good effect. this became a great favorite with the men, all asking for

---

335 "*De temporibus anni insalubribus*" ("Of unhealthful seasons of the year"): Hoffmann, *Opera omnia*, V, sect. i, cap. v, pp. 63–9. Hoffmann asserts that bad air causes illness; that the west wind is most healthful; and that dry air is usually most salubrious.

336 "*De siderum in corpora humana influxu medico*" ("Of sidereal influence on the human body"): ibid., cap. vi, pp. 70–6. Although this dissertation, which originally was published at Halle in 1706, appears in Hoffmann's collected works, the author was Johann Andreas Usenbenz. In his dissertation, Usenbenz argues that while it is necessary for medical men to reject astrology and superstition, the sun and moon clearly influence human health and body rhythms.

337 Hippocrates, Affections, c.29.

338 Hippocrates, Internal Affections, c.51.

339 Ibid.

302. [*facing p. 301; blank*]

303. [*continuing on from p. 301*]:
the little black pill, saying, it <does> them a deale of good & was worth it's weight in gold. None of the Officers had complaints of this kind, but it was common with their Servants, being more exposed to the injuries of the weather. Many men were seized on Duty viz: the grand Guard &c: this continued to the end of the Campn. & the above method seldom failed of Success.

{**"I used to think that the practice of medicine in camps had peculiar features very different from what one observes in cities, and that it was so abnormal and irregular that one had to snatch at what remedies were to be had and apply them with a certain rashness."**} Ramaz: de morb: Artif. Cap:42.[340] [**he says,**}

{**"Men spend so short a part of their life in camp that it seemed to me that their medical treatment ought not to demand too much time but be prompt and offhand; that in proportion as the emergency itself is urgent, any experiments must involve risks; that is, in short, a doctor, however willing, could not on account of unforeseen accidents and the constant shifting of a camp, undertake a regular course of treatment, any more than his patient could .... Many distinguished men perished because the doctors, who knew nothing of military medicine or the peculiar character of camp diseases, prescribed for them ill-chosen remedies such as venesection and strong purgatives."**}[341]

[*margin:* Leeches applyed to the joints.] in obstinate Rheumatisms with swelled joints I have known Leeches applyed to the part, with such good success that the Patients often desire to have them renewed. in the hospital this form is much used as a Sudorificke, {**Take equal quantities of *vinum emeticum*, *tinctura antimonii*, and *spiritus cornu cervi*; mix an electuary; 80 to 100 drops.**} with warm posset drink[.] this Desease is the certaine attendant of a late Campn. when the Evenings grow long, yet the weather may be pleasant, tho cold; & mo<o>nshine invite to walk abroad, rather than sit confined to

304. [*facing p. 303; blank*]

305. [*continuing from p. 303*]:

---

340 Ramazzini, *De morbis artificum* (trans. Wright), p. 361.

341 Ibid., pp. 361, 375.

a small tent: at this time the dews fall heavie, the grass is damp, & the Summer cloaths are yet worn, & by this time our tents are wore thin & tore, raine & damps passing easely thro them[a].

[*margin:* Westbaden bath.] in the neighbourhood of our Camp in Germany was a famous warm Bath for Gouty & Rheumatic limbs &c: viz: at Westbaden. The water comes smoaking hot from the Spring with a strong Sulphureous smell, boyling like a Copper, so hot that I durst not keep my finger in it the least moment of time, nor touch it with my toes for fear of scalding. it's said to be hot enough to harden an egg in five minutes, & will codle Apples &c: tastes of a Strong Sea Salt & Sulphur. is drunk to two pots in a morning & purges briskly. is said to be good for all deseases of old age; many Rheumatick & Gouty patients were bathing, cupping &c: Some Officers & Soldiers bathed on account of Stiff joints from Gunshot wounds & received great benefit.

{**"And some parts of him, still warm with life, he boiled."**}
Ov: Met: lib:i. V:228.[342]

& here I received immedeate relief for a swelled knee which had continued upwards of Six weeks, & threatned a stiff joint, was occasioned by a horse falling with me in the Streets of Mayence. I was much refreshed by bathing. the water seems to be of a stronger body than that of Aix la chapelle, for my body could hardly sink in it. cold water is brought in by pipes to make it what heat You please.

[*margin:* Lumbago Rheumatica.] Many had Lumbago Rheumatica[,] could not stand upright[;] were rubed with Lint. vol: covering with flannel; when in hospital, were blistered, or issues cut.

We tooke the field May 19th N:S: 1744. and

306.
{**"The sun should be avoided and the cool of morning and evening and whatever breezes come from rivers, pools, and snow."**} Hip: de vict: rat: lib.2.[343]
vid: Philippus Weberus, Thermarum Wisbadensium descriptio. Oppenheimi 1617. 4[to.344]

307. [*continuing from p. 305*]:
encamped on a wet Soyle amongst ranke corn; the weather cold & wet.

---

342 Ovid, Metamorphoses, 1.228–9. This quotation is drawn from Jupiter's account of an attempt by Lycaon to deceive him into eating human flesh.

343 Hippocrates, Regimen, c.68.

344 Philipp Weber, *Thermarum Wisbadensium descriptio. Complectens antiquitatem et utilitatem harum thermarum* (Oppenheim: Hieronymi Galleri, 1617). Weber discusses the antiquity of the baths, the quality and mineral component of the waters, the illnesses and infirmities that they relieve, and regimen for bathers. He sees the baths as a virtual panacea.

[*margin:* Deases (*sic*) in Camp. 1744.] Agues & Quincies, with slight aching pains were frequent. at first taking the field it's common to have many kicks from the horses, being then in great heart & full of play. Slight wounds do not Suppurate so well as in Garrison, should be keep'd warmer with flannel &c: On leaving Garrison the men & Servants are apt to get drink over night in taking leave of their Landlords, &c. & we have many accidents. nixt day & much confusion in passing the Gates. attended with many inconveniences, carriages are overturned, broke down, men hurt & horses lamed.

> {**"The maddened horses leap apart, wrench their necks from the yoke, and break away from the parted reins. Here lie the reins, there the axle torn from the pole; in another place the spokes of the broken wheels, and fragments of the wrecked chariot are scattered far and wide."**}
>
> Ov: met: lib:ii. V:314.[345]
>
> {**"But Phaethon ... is hurled headlong [and falls with a long trail through the air]."**}
>
> V.388.[346]

When the weather become dry & warm, the ground dry, Complaints were much the same as last Season, but having little or no fatigue, the weather was not so excessive hot, they were neither so frequent nor violent. The men were accustomed to a Campn life, were always supplyed with plenty of good provision, abundance of Straw, lived well & made huts to shed themselves from the Sun, which we never did in Germany on account of frequent marching, nor did the Country afford such plenty of wood, nor durst we make free with it as in Flanders.

308. [*facing p. 307; blank*]

309. [*continuing on from p. 307*]:

> {**"This abode is a second home for the soldier, its rampart takes the place of city walls and his own tent is the soldier's dwelling and hearthside."**}
>
> Liv: xliv.99.[347]

Speaking of the Roman encampments & Caesar observes in lib:3 of the civile wars,

{**"[In the camp of Pompeius ...] huts ... of Lucius Lentulus and some others [were] covered over with ivy."**}[348]

---

[345] Ovid Met. 2.314–18.

[346] Ibid., 2.319, 320.

[347] Livy, 44.39.5.

[348] Caesar, Civil Wars, 3.96.

{"This retreat, so sweet – yes, believe me, so bewitching – keeps me, my friend, in sound health in September's heat."}

Hor: Ep:16. lib:1.[349]

{"… their lord with plenteous shade."}.

Ib: Ep.17: lib:i.[350]

{"Is there any where winters are milder, where a more grateful breeze tempers the Dog-star's fury and the Lion's onset, when once in frenzy he has caught the sun's piercing shafts?"}

Ep.x. lib:i.[351]

{"Here in retired valley shalt thou escape the dog-star's heat."}

Od:17. lib:i. V:17. &c:[352]

{"Thee the fierce season of the blazing dog-star cannot touch."}

Od:13. lib:3tis.[353]

[*margin:* the Regiment remarkably healthie in Campn 1744.] Our men drunk freely, eating all sorts of Summer fruits in abundance, yet there was not the least appearance of fluxes; the whole army remarkablie healthie. July 30th the return of Genll Cope's Regmt of Dragoons amounted to only Nine Sicke & Lame & all triffling Cases. the first man I sent to the hospital was Robinson of Sr James's, being lately recovered a slight fever, & so weake that he was unfit to march. July 31st. When at Anstaine Camp the Hospital was fix't at Tournay, & preparations being made for fifty Sicke, twenty were ordered to be sent from the Cavalry & thirty from the infantry. the Cavalry sent but Sixteen tho we were three Regmts of horse, Six of Dragoons, & three troops of horse Guards.

{"Many delight in the camp, in the sound of the trumpet mingled with the clarion, and in the wars that mothers hate."}

Hor: Od:i. lib:i[a].[354]

about the latter end of Augst. our Duty began to be very hard and

310.

[a]Desertion was the most prevailing distemper, & thought to proceed from the inactivity of our Army; all nations equally subject to it, but more especially the Irish. it was not known amongst the horse, their pay was too good to run away from: nor was there any such thing amongst the Highlanders, being ashamed of their great desertion

---

349 Horace, Epistles, 1.16.15–16.

350 Ibid., 1.17.10.

351 Ibid., 1.10.15–17.

352 Horace, Odes, 1.17.17–18.

353 Ibid., 3.13.9–10.

354 Ibid., 1.1.23–5.

on coming over. mild remedies were at first tryed viz: wheeping, but not proving succesfull, & the desease growing dayly more desperate, desperate remedies must be put in practice, & hanging was the only Specifick. the Romans punished desertion with great Severity. C: Matienus had quitted the army in Spain without a discharge. he was accused for this reason befor the tribunes, & by their Sentence condemned to be whipped with the *Furca* (or Gibbet) on his neck, & afterwards to be sold for the lowest price, (*Sestertio nummo.* about three half pence) as being of less value than the meanest of Slaves. this Sentence was executed in the presence of the new raised Soldiers the Consuls were then levying. Roll. Rom: hist. V:8th.[355]

311. [*continuing on from p. 309*]:
fatiguing from out parties, forraging, &c: the covering party for forraging turning out at break of day, & the forragers an hour or two thereafter. worke hard all day in cutting corn, mowing Grass, making trusses &c: and don't return till evening; the old Grand Guard is often employed on this duty, are thirty or forty hours a horsebacke, & often without forrage. we sometimes went fifteen miles in search of forrage, (which at home would be reckoned a long march) & return with heavie trusses, the men mounted. Some parties were ordered out over night, in order to cover the forragers nixt day, were obliged to lye on their arms in the open field, stand to their arms all nixt day, & return to Camp at night & often wet to the skine, & some accidents of Gunshot wounds from skirmishing with the Enemies out parties[a].

[*margin:* The Regmt sickly from much fatigue.] then Sicknes began, & September 6th my Return was Bloody fluxes three, Agues 6. Fevers nine; Rheumatisms two, Venereals five, Surgery cases Six, Sick & Lame in the hospital eight.

[*margin:* Officers healthy.] the Officers all in good health, neither Sick not Lame during this Camp.

{"No cough or pleurisy or gout [would kill Horace]."}
Hor.[356]

[*penciled vertical line in margin next to the following*]
Spare dyet with good exercise & light wines seems to be the best preservative from Distempers. their constant Dyet was green tea with bread & butter for breakfast. Soupe with plaine boyled or roasted meats for Dinner, drinking Burgundy or Spanish mountaine[,] bread & cheese or some slight thing for Supper, with a Glas wine in moderation & were merry over their Cups. Many lose their bellies being obliged to shorten their sword belts & take in the west band

355 Rollin, *Roman History*, VIII, 256; "had quitted … levying" is quoted.
356 Horace, Satires, 1.9.32.

312.

[a] **{"For many days [Ceres] tarried motionless under the open sky, patiently enduring the moonlight and the rain."}**

Ov: fast: lib:4. V.505.[357]

{"Not a place but has its own peculiar destiny."}[358]

313. [*continuing on from p. 312*]:

of their breeches, & think themselves some Stones lighter, being every way more active & nimble.

{"Nights of vigil make thin the bodies of lovers, and anxiety and the distress that a great passion brings."}

Ov: art: Amat: lb:ii. V:737.[359]

[*margin:* health or Sickness greatly depend on the weather.] During this Campn I keep't an exact journal of the weather from a small Thermometer, as to heat or cold, wet or dry; and accordingly observed my return of Sick & Lame, rise & fall like a weather Glas.

[*margin:* horses healthie in Camp.] Our horses were healthie eating all sorts of green forrage, & that without any bad consequence, tho some dyed, & said to be from over-eating. the men were carefull in feeding sparingly & mixing some dry forrage with the green. feeding with Rye when full in the Ear, gives a sore mouth, so that they can neither eat oates nor dry forrage, the Groome should be carefull in cleaning his mouth. as they had little or no fatigue they were exceedingly fat & in fine order.

[*margin:* horses much affected by change of weather.] it's surprising how suddenly this creature is affected by the change of weather. all were in fine order Septr 9th but that night being cold & frosty wind, their coats stared nixt morning as if it had been the midle of winter, which continued during this Campn.

[*margin:* horses suffer much from fatigue in Camp.] Many had sore backs being bruised from carrying heavie trusses; the common method of cure is applying warm Dung & covering with a thick horse cloth, some use blacke Soape & brandy[a]. Some were sprained across the Loins, not able to walke & never able to carry a weight; the cure is attempted by Strengthening plaisters or charges, first rubbing with warm oils, some

314.

[a] the German servants make use of the juice of the long leaved plantane, if the skin was broke; covering the part with the leave, & proved a good dryer and healer.

---

357 Ovid, Fasti, 4.505–6.

358 Ibid., 4.507.

359 Ovid, Art of Love, 1.735–6.

315. [*continuing on from p. 313*]:
cover with a Sheep's skin newly taken from the beast, but it requires long time & much rest; Such as did not recover to carry burdens were employed as draught horses nixt Campn. Some were shoulder slip't were blooded & oyled, rowelled &c: few recovered as Troop horses, but did well enough to go at a foot's pace in a plough or cart. Complaints of this kind were frequent by the latter end of the Campn from the great fatigue of forraging. Some horses dyed on the road, others had their backs broke & were shot as useless.

> {**"The horse, once of high courage and of great renown on the race course, has now lost his victorious spirit and, forgetting his former glory, groans in his stall, doomed to an inglorious death .... Lethargy holds all. In woods and fields and roads foul carcasses lie; and the air is defiled by the stench."**}
> Ov: met: lb:7. V:542.[360]

[*margin:* hair rubed off their huckle bones.] few escaped having the hair rubed off their huckle bones & other parts from carrying trusses.

> {**"[Horace may ride a mule,] the saddle-bag's weight galling his loins, and the rider his withers."**}
> Hor: Sat:5. lb:i.[361]

this Oynt. was recommended by my Lord Albemarle[362] in order to make the hair grow in 24 hours. Rx. hogs lard lb.i. Turpentine, St. John's wort, Assafoetida aa oz.i. make into an Oynt. Many horse Officers mark'd it in their pocket books, but I never remember any thing of its good effect. it seems to be rather commanding than assisting Nature, and puts me in mind of what Dioscorides says of the Vitex or Agnus Castus. viz: being held in the hand it preserveth the Rider from galling, which must have been a valuable Recepe, especially as Saddles were scarcely in fashion in his time[363a].

316. [*margin:* Crib-biting horses.] there's a great affinity 'twixt the deseases of men & horses,
but I don't know any desease incident to the humane body resembling the crib-biting in horses, unless it be the custome of children sucking their fingers. the horse takes a fancy to bite the Manger, picket or picket roape, pinching & squeezing with his teeth, making a grunting noise, & straining hard with the muscles of his neck, as if convulsed; by frequent biting they

---

360 Ovid, Metamorphoses, 7.542–4, 547–8.

361 Horace, Satires, 1.6[not 5].106.

362 William Anne Keppel, 2nd earl of Albemarle (1702–54).

363 "The seeds thereof being smeared on with water, do lessify the chaps in ye seate"; Dioscorides, *The Greek Herbal of Dioscorides*, trans. John Goodyer, ed. Robert T. Gunther (Oxford: Oxford Univ. Press, 1934), p. 74.

wear away the foreteeth, lick often with their tongue & suck in wind at the same time filling their belly so full that they are in danger of bursting. are in great pain & agony, the body being much swelled, rolling and tumbling about. the Farriers bleed in the mouth, & racke, giving a drink of some warm seeds in order to breake wind & scower thro them. this is infectious, for he who Crib:bites learns his nixt neighbour to do the same. We therefor make such horses stand by themselves, driving their picket so close to the ground, that they cannot catch hold of it; yet they often snap & catch hold of the collar, & this they often attemp [*sic*] even when blind. some naile a Sheep's taile or greasie wool to the manger, or picket, & the horse does not touch it, & some tye a broad Strap round the horse's neck, as tight as he can bear it, which prevents their sucking wind, & breaks them of that custome.

317. [*continuing on from p. 315*]:

[*margin:* English horses much tormented by the flies, for want of their taile.] English horses for want of their tails are greatly tormented with flies during the warm weather; fatigue themselves with kicking & stamping, wear out their Shoes, breake & Spoyle the ground; tossing their heads backwards to beat off the flies, lose their forrage. the fatigue is so much that it makes them sweat as they stand at the picket, & fall off their flesh. None of our Allies docke their horses & are allowed a smaller <u>ratiate</u> than ours, by two or three pounds of hay, yet are fatter & look better than ours by the latter end of the Campn.; their Masters are more carefull in cutting wheat Straw & mixing with their oates, which fills their bellies & keeps them healthfull, whilst we throw the Straw befor our horses uncut, which is trampled into the ground & lost.

[*margin:* very bad weather at the latter end of Campn 1744.] Septr 29th N:S. we decamped from Anstaine camp, had violent rains, high winds, & cold weather during the remaining part of the Campn.

{**"The morning frosts are nipping now, if people are careless."**}
Hor: Sat:6. lb.2. V:45.[364]

& tho encamped near Ghent we were in want of provision, the weather being so very bad, none of the inhabitants could come to Camp. Some tents were tore to pieces, & some could not be pitched on account of the high winds. the men & their accoutrements were so wet as to be unfit for duty. the horses starving with cold & hunger.

{**"Not for ever will my body endure thy threshold or the rain of heaven."**}
Hor: Od:10. lb:iii. V.19.[365]

During this weather the Officers sat in the Sutlers tent night &

364 Horace, Satires, 2.6.45.
365 Horace, Odes, 3.10.19–20.

318. [*facing p. 317; blank*]

319. [*continuing on from p. 317]*:
day, tho almost tore to pieces & the ground wet under foot. yet none catched cold, all bearing well, laughing at each others misfortunes, & taking a cheerful Glas.

> {**"Then, as night comes on, let them steep themselves in wine."**}
>
> Hor: Sat:1. lb:ii. V:9.[366]
>
> [**"Nor are cankering cares dispelled except by Bacchus' gift. Who, after his wine, harps on the hardships of campaigns or poverty? Who does not rather glorify thee, O Father Bacchus, and thee, O comely Venus? And yet, that no one pass the bounds of moderation in enjoying Liber's gifts, we have a lesson in the Centaurs' contest with the Lapithae, fought out to the bitter end over the festal board."**}
>
> Hor: Od:18. lib:1. V:3.[367]

but in England had any one of them lodged in a room lately washed, it must have been well aired, & the bed warmed; here were noe complaints, all bearing their misfortunes with great patience.

> {**"Do the eagerness, pray, and delight that men have in hunting carry them through snow and frost into the mountains and the forests; and shall not we use in the stress of war the same resolution which even sport and pleasure are wont to call out?"**} Liv: lib:5.[368]

Cpt. Gilbert did not put off his cloaths for nineteen nights, always laye on Straw in his Servants tent; yet had no complaints tho a delicate man.

> {**"[A free man is one who] scorns ambition [and] in himself is a whole, smoothed and rounded."**}.
>
> Hor:[369]

The Dutch & Hanoverians kep't the field ten days after us, the weather continuing wet & cold, the whole country flooded. & tho I imagined we could stand it no longer, yet I don't remember to hear of an extraordinary sickness amongst them. it's surprizing what people can do when forced to it. many tender women & young children marched

320. [*facing p. 319; blank*]

321. [*continuing on from p. 319*]:

---

366 Horace, Satires, 2.1.9.

367 Horace, Odes, 1.18.3–9.

368 Livy, 5.6.3.

369 Horace, Satires, 2.7.85–6.

with us last year thro Germany, were never a horseback, nor carried in waggons. at Windsor Forest Camp, children of eight years old marched from Glasgow to that Camp in a month's time[a]. One of our Troopers wifes in Germany marched 36 hours with the child in her arms, the fourth day after delivery.

> **{"In her arms she [i.e. Dryope] bore a pleasing burden, her infant boy not yet a full year old, and nursed him at her breast."}**
>
> Ov: met: lib:9. V.359.[370]

[*margin:* Deseases in Camp. 1745.] We took the field April 30th N:S: 1745. encamping on good dry ground. tho a short march, we had much fatigue; were mounted at four in the morning, but did not come to our ground till near Sunset, & our baggage did not come up till ten at night[x]. The beginning of May was wet & cold. Quincies & Rheumaticke complaints, & grieps threatning a flux, were common. as we approached near the Enemy, we had great fatigue from advanced Posts, Grand Guards &c: & complaints were much the same as befor the battle of Dettenghen.

after the action of Fontenoye the Sick & wounded were sent to the Hospital at Ath, the Soldiers barracks being fitted up for that purpose, & are the most commodious we have yet had, each apartment containing only Six or Seven beds, a proper fire place, are well aired, & each roome seperated by a wall, & our sicke recovered well.[371] it's a general fault in all hospitals, that the apartments are too large, & containe too many sicke, by which the air is infected, especially in warm weather, & when the house is crowded after an action[a].

Octr 1st I was ordered to attend a party from Vilfort to Mons, which continued fourteen days, tho we did not expect it would have lasted half that time, & of course

322.

[a] **{"Let it gather strength by experiencing; so but you nurture it well, in time it will**

---

[370] Ovid, Metamorphoses, 9.338–9. Soldiers' wives and children seldom travelled in wagons, except when seriously ill: Paul E. Kopperman, "The British High Command and Soldiers' Wives in America, 1755–1783," *Journal of the Society for Army Historical Research*, 60 (1982), pp. 29, 30n56.

[371] According to Pringle, about 600 wounded were sent to the facility at Ath, which was opened the day after the battle. It remained in service until 25 Aug., in all treating 991 patients, of whom 59 died, a low percentage compared to other hospital bases and especially impressive given that some of the patients had been seriously wounded at Fontenoy. H. A. L. Howell, "The Story of the Army Surgeon and the Care of the Sick and Wounded in the British Army, from 1715 to 1748." *Journal of the Royal Army Medical Corps*, 22 (1914), p. 458; Pringle, *Observations on the Diseases*, p. 35.

be strong".}

Ov.[372]

[x]the men of most distinction of Philip of Macedon's army were not permitted to make use of any carrages in their march, either for themselves or their baggage; which was allowed to be no more than their Servants could carry: nor were the number of these permitted to be any greater than strict necessity required. Leland's history of the life & reign of Philip King of Macedon. one of his Officers was dismissed from his service for using warm Baths, & two others for entertaining a singing Girl. Ib Vol. 1st. their wives were never suffered to attend his Officers. Ib.[373]

[a.]feverish complaints were common after the battle, the day was very hot, & great fatigue, some being fourty hours a horseback. large bleeding the best remedy. with rest[x.] and opiates. with some those fevers continued a long while, from the great concern of the mind only*, nor could they refraine from talking of the action. were sometimes delirious, & talked of Entrenchements, Dispositions, Batteries &c: I blooded Coll F: twice in less than ½ an hour's time. & it was necessary to bleed his Royale Highness[374] by way of prevention.

{"He whom reason, not anger, animates is a peer of the gods."}

Claudianus.[375]

{"[Aeneas] his heart troubled by woeful war, stretched him on the bank under the sun's chill cope, and let late sleep steal over his limbs."}

Virg: – vid: L'art de conserver la Sante de Princes &c par Cornaro.[376]

***{"He [Jupiter] conceived a mighty wrath worthy of the soul of Jove."}**

Ov:[377]

[x.]**{"O Sleep, thou rest of all things, Sleep, mildest of the Gods, balm of the soul, who puttest care to flight, soothest our bodies worn with hard ministries, and preparest them for toil again."}**

---

372 Ovid, Art of Love, 2.339–40.

373 Thomas Leland, *The Life and Reign of Philip King of Macedon, the Father of Alexander*, 2nd ed. (London: E. Johnston, 1775), I, 79; "the men … required," "one officer was dismissed … singing girl," and "their wives … his officers;" are all quoted passages.

374 i.e., Cumberland; "Coll. F." was presumably Col. Robert Fraser of the 3rd (Scots) Foot Guards, who was wounded at Fontenoy; note Townshend's return: C. V. F. Townshend, *The Military Life of FieldMarshal George First Marquess Townshend 1724–1807* (London: John Murray, 1901), p. 77.

375 Claudian, "Panegyric on the Consulship of Manlius," 227–8.

376 Virgil, Aeneid, 8.29–30. This passage is also quoted in *L'art de conserver*, p. 207.

377 Ovid, Metamorphoses, 1.166.

Ov:[378]

323. [*continuing on from p. 321*]:
made little or no preparation for such an expedition, marching with as little baggage as possible. we had great fatigue, marching night & day, horses stood Saidled three or four days. the men often without Straw, & one night without their tents[c.]. having so much duty there was no time to provide victuals, ammonition bread was their chief food, & sometimes obliged to drink muddy water with their horses. being always in boots, there were many swelled legs. the weather was cold, frosty, but dry, & there was no great Sickness. slight Rheumaticks & sore throats the chief complaints.

[*margin:* great fatigue on out parties.] few officers had any bedding, & some never put off their cloaths[b.]; cooked what they could most easely find[d.], were healthfull & cheerfull all the while.

{"Night, storm, long journeys, cruel pains, all kinds of toil are in this dainty camp. Oft will you put up with rain from melting clouds of heaven, and oft will you cold lie on the bare ground."}

Ov: art: amat: lib:ii. V:234[a.].[379]

The Highland Regmt marched in our front, some had sprained anckles & sore feet. they were in high Spirits, & stood the March well. the Prince of Waldeck's Regmt of Grenadiers brought up the rear, a most beautefull Regmt & remarkable for their large size; were greatly fatigued & much ado to reach camp, many dropping on the March.

{"Such as inhabit a region that is mountainous, rugged, high, and poorly watered, and the seasons of the year exhibit sharp contrasts, are likely to be big, with a nature well adapted for toil and vigor, and such have not a little brutality and wildness."} Hip: de Aere, locis et Aqua.[380]

if we continue

324.

[c.] **{"That which lacks its alternations of repose will not endure; this is what repairs the strength and renews the wearied limbs."}**

Ov: Ep:4. V:89.[381]

[b.] **{"We reposed beneath the sheltering trees, where mingled grass and leaves afforded us a couch."}**

---

[378] Ibid., 11.623–5.

[379] Ovid, Art of Love, 2.235–8.

[380] Hippocrates, Air, Places, Water, c.24.

[381] Ovid, Heroides, 4.89–90.

Ov: Ep:5. V.13.[382]

[d.] **{"Woodland was their home, their food grass, their bedding leaves."}**

Ov:[383]

[a.] **{"I, who once shunned affairs, who was born for a care-free life of ease, who was soft and incapable of toil, am now suffering extremes .... And my spirit has proved equal to misfortune; for my body, borrowing strength from that spirit, has endured things scarce endurable."}**

Ov: tris: lib:iii. V:91.[384]

325. [*continuing on from p. 323*]:
long in one Camp our <men> grow lousy & itchy.

[*margin:* some inconveniences from encamping too long in the same ground.] their straw should be often changed; the old always burnt & not thrown as litter to the horses. the men have much ado to keep their long hair free from vermine, & it's a custom with them to anoint their hair with Ungt. Mercurial instead of Pomatum, & kill vermine of all sorts. some use an Oynt. of red precipitate one pennyworth mixed with butter, Ryslie of Cpt. Loyd's used it often, but catching cold in the wet weather in the latter end of Campn 1744 got into a high Salivation, & with difficulty was purged off. if we remaine a long time in the same Camp, there's an ugly smell, from the horse Dung, & large swarms of flies become troublesome, especially in hot weather. if the ground be wettish, with many ditches of stagnating water, fish ponds, &c: the water stinks in hot weather & is useless, being full of frogs Spawn &c: Fabius the Roman General said, that it was not for the advantage of an army to continue always or long in the same place: that marching & change rendered it fitter for action, & contributed to the health of the Soldier. Roll: Rom: Hist:[385]

{"I must change my resort, and drive my horse past the familiar lodgings."}

Hor: Ep:15. lib:1. V:10.[386]

[*margin:* The Dog days.] people look for much sickness about the Dog days & expect excessive heats; but I have not observed any particular sickness at this time.

---

[382] Ibid., 5.13–14.

[383] Ovid, Art of Love, 2.475.

[384] Ovid, Tristia, 3.2.9–11, 13–14.

[385] *Roman History*, III, 246; "said … soldiers" is quoted. The passage refers to Fabius Rullianus Maximus, and action in 295 b.c.e.

[386] Horace, Epistles, 1.15.10–11.

{"There is a Dog (they call it the Icarian dog), and when that constellation rises the earth is parched and dried, and the crop ripens too soon."}

Ov: fast: lib:5. V:939.[387]

in hot weather the men are too much clothed, especially when fully accoutred & mounted with all their baggage, & some faint under the

326. [*facing p. 325; blank*]

327. [*continuing on from p. 325*]:
Burden, & others from real fatigue & long fasting[a.]. common custom calls out for bleeding immediately, & that without Ryme or Reason. I order them to have the free use of the coole refreshing air, & to be laid at full length, giving a little wine by way of cordial. if from a Plethora, bleeding is then necessary & a Glas of water the best Cordiale. When the men find themselves faint & spent, they imagine bleeding might relieve them & beg to be blooded, but I rather advise them to compose themselves to rest, refreshing themselves with wine & bread rubed with Nutmeg &c:

{"In cardiac disease the one hope of relief lies undoubtedly in wine."}

Plin: lib:22.[388]

[*margin:* Convulsive fitts.] Convulsive Fits proceed from passions of the mind. Mercer of Cpt. Loyds's is often subject to them on being drunk or vexed; he has acted sometime as Depute-Corporale & expected being appointed full Corpll on the first vacancy, but was put by, & greatly disappointed; fell into a violent fit, & continued near two hours, strugling so hard that four of his Comrades could scarcely hold him, he endeavoured to bite everything, his tongue often in danger, but was prevented by putting a <u>tent-pin</u> across his mouth. I give Op: in large doses & compose them to sleep. Smith of the King's Troop, took Laud: Liquid gt.120 & upon recovery found himself greatly refreshed, whereas at other times he always complained of great soreness about the breast. Jeffard of Capt. Shipman's is a very irregular fellow, often drunk, & is often ordered to be picketted; but so soon as he is mounted, falls into violent convulsive fitts, & by this means escapes punishment. I have often given him fourscore drops Laudanum.

{"No one dares to give southernwood to the sick unless he has learned its use."}

---

[387] Ovid, Fasti, 4(not 5).939–40.

[388] Pliny, Natural History, 23[not 22].25.50. cf. above, n. 56. Discounting the quotation from Catullus that is in one case smudged (n. 125), this is the only case in which Buchanan quotes the same passage twice.

Hor: Ep.i. lib:ii. V:114b.[389]

328.

a. the old & wore out men are dayly subject to complaints of this kind; rest & nourishing dyet the only medecine.

{"... old as he [i.e. Priam] is, he vainly throws his long-disused armour about his aged trembling shoulders, girds on his useless sword ...."}

Vir: Aen:2. V:509.[390]

b. [*margin:* Apoplexy] Apoplecticks are blooded largely, purged briskly, blistered &c: ordered to live sparingly & abstaine from drinking. are most frequent on long marching & hot weather, fatigue &c: our troopers cloathing are too heavie for the Summer, especially when fully accoutred & mounted with all their baggage, some faint under the burthen. it's commonly said the third Apoplectick fit carries off the Patient; but I have known Carter of Cpt. Gilbert's have many, as also Maynard of the King's.

329. [*continuing on from p. 327*]:

[*margin:* Melancholy.] Soldiers sometimes take a melancholy turn, become lowe spirited, senseless & childish, avoid company, cry or mutter to themselves, love to be solitary. upon asking their case, they tell long stories about their past & present condition, are in great fear of being some way or other lost. such as make hasty resolutions of abstaining from all sorts of strong liquors, to which they were formerly accustomed, are most subject to this complaint, & those who have been disappointed of their due preferment, nor is there any end of their complaints & of the injustice done them after so long service. Vomits & exercise are the chief medecines, but a heartie bottle gives present relief.

{"There are spells and sayings whereby you may soothe the pain and cast much of the malady aside."}

Hor: Ep:1. lib:1.[391]

---

389 Horace, Epistles, 2.1.114–15.

390 Virgil, Aeneid, 2.509–11.

391 Horace, Epistles, 1.1.34.

& to make it more medicinal I order pil: Assafoetid.[392] to be taken two or three times a day, & washed down with a Glass of wine[x], <[x]Pechlin: obs: Med: lib.3 no.16.[393]> & advise cheerfull company.

> **{"If alone, you will be sad .... And fly not intercourse, nor let your door be closed, nor hide your tearful countenance in darkness."}**
>
> Ov: rem: Am: V:585.[394]

Some are so morose & sulkie in their tempers that they will not be perswaded to take anything, much ado to prevaile on them to eat or drinke. I endeavour to make them merry by putting wine into their Soupe &c[.]

> **{"By his eloquence he [i.e. Ajax] will calm the hero [i.e. Philoctetes], mad with pain and rage, or else by some shrewd trick will bring him to us."}**
>
> Ov: met: lb:13. V:322.[395]
>
> vid: L'Eloge de Lyvresse[a].[396]

[*margin:* Drunkards healthie.] The Drunken fellows have been remarkably healthie since we came abroad; the same was observed in the late West Indian expedition, the Drunken fellows only lived to come home:

330.

[*margin:* Deafnes.] [a]Many complain of deafnes from catching cold by lying on the wet ground, or on being long confined at the Provoes. the ears are Syringed in hopes of bring out some wax, oyle being first poured in, in order to soften or loosen it. the common method of Syringing the ears with a small Syringe is good for nothing; there not being a sufficient quantity of water injected at one time to soften the wax; I therefor use a large clyster Syringe, nor does there appear any danger in breaking the Tympanum, having tryed as much force as could be applyed to this Syringe in injecting the ears of a dead person, yet the Tympanum not in

---

392 There was no official "asafetida pill." *Practice* lists two nervine pills that include asafetida, "gum pills" and "nervous pills": *Practice of the British and French Hospitals*, pp. 67, 68.

393 Pechlin's chapter (*Observationum*, III, no. xvi, pp. 432–5) is entitled, "Morbus imaginarius" ("Imaginary illness" or "Illness caused by the imagination"). In it, he states the importance of treating the patient's mind as well as body and of using deceit when necessary to "cure" an imagined illness.

394 Ovid, Cure for Love, v.583, 587–8.

395 Ovid, Metamorphoses, 13.322–3.

396 *L'Eloge de L'Yvresse*, by Albert Henri de Sallengre (La Haye: Pierre Gosse, 1714). In citing this work, Buchanan may have had in mind particularly chs. 2–3 ("That *Wine* drives away Sorrow and excites Mirth"; "That it is good for one's health to get drunk sometimes").

the least hurt. Soap & water is my injection, & has often succeeded in bringing out hard wax & some cotton which was introduced some years ago, & become hard as a Stone. this method was tryed with Ashberry of Majr. Jenkinson's, but without any good effect; his deafnes was suspected by his Comrades, as a pretence to obtaine his discharge & had the desired effect; & they say, he recovered his hearing as he returned home.

[a.] {**Treatment of someone maddened by love: "Occasionally also he must be diverted to other interests, disquietudes, cares, occupations; finally he is frequently curable by change of scene as is done with sick people who are slow in making recovery."**} Cic: Thus: l:5.[397]

{**"A Passion of the Mind is not to be conquered by Medicine, but by some contrary Passion. Anger and Hope remove Fear, and Joy takes away Sorrow."**} Sanct: Aph: 4 C7.[398]

331. [*continuing on from p. 329*]:
but when taken ill, their distempers are more violent, & some dye suddenly[x]. Vid. Carr. Epist: Medic: No. 4.[399] Chapman of Captn. Gilberts dyed suddenly in the hospital, as he was recovering a violent fever, & was ready to be discharged, but was suddenly seized with an acute pain in the upper & inside of the left thigh, saying it came like a shot of a Gun, & that it was so violent that it would certainly kill him; the part was neither swelled nor discoloured, nor any thing observable to the touch, tho fomented & poulticed, found no relief; continued in great Agony that night, next morning said he could bear it no longer, that he was sure to dye, drunk a dish <of> Coffee, & dyed presently. the thigh swelled a little by nixt morning, was of a livid colour. in the affected part there was much ichorose-gelatinous-jelly, & the appearance of a beginning mortification, tho no deeper than the cellular Substance. Quaer: 1mo. was this an attempt of nature to form a criticale absess here. 2do. would scarifications with warm digestives been of any use.

[*margin:* Dissection of a Drunkard.] Upon dissecting the body all the cartilages of the ribs were strongly ossified, were cut with chizel & mallet[;] all the bowels remarkably sound & in good order, no dry or burnt liver as is said to be the case with Drunkards, & was probably owing to his drinking malt liquor rather than Gin.

---

397 Cicero, Tusculan Disputations, 4.74.

398 *Medicina statica*, p. 306.

399 Richard Carr, *Dr. Carr's Medicinal Epistles Upon Several Occasions: Done into English, as a Supplement to the Explanations of Sanctorious's Aphorisms*, trans. John Quincy (London: William Newton and J. Phillips, 1714), pp. 31–9; cf. Carr, *Epistolae medicinales variis occasionibus conscriptae* (London: Stafford Anson, 1691), pp. 36–46.

[*margin:* Deseases on coming into Garrison.] After coming into Garrison many have coughs, & feverish disorders with aching pains, &c: from catching cold in the latter end of the Campn, & are treated accordingly. it's observed many people fall ill on their coming from Camp, & some Officers who are carefull of preserving

332.

[x] {**"… seeing that hope is disappointed now and again, and that the patient dies whom the practitioner at first deemed safe; and further that measures proper for curing now and again make a change into something worse. Nor, in the face of such a variety of temperaments, can human frailty avoid this."**} Cels: lib:2. C:vi.[400]

Tissot on Bilious fevers. has much such an other case of a Young fellow, afflicted with a most violent pain in the left arm, p. i09 [*sic*].[401]

333. [*continuing on from p. 331*]:
health, endeavour to live at their first coming into Garrison, in the same manner they did in Camp, or as near to it as possible. tho a fire in the roome, they seldome sit near it, nor do they air a shirt, walk a foot in the dirty street. those who are of a sedentary disposition are most subject to be taken ill; they were healthie during the Campn. from being much on their legs & moving about, by the latter end of the Season the field began to be tyresome to them & wished heartely for Winter Quarters, where they shut themselves up in their rooms, indulging in bed[a] or loitering in an easie chair, taking to their books & study, not caring to stir abroad, saying, they have had enough of that lately. from this sudden change they become heavie & dull, lowspirited, their appetite failes, grow sicklie & unactive; then bleed, vomite, & take bitters, & unjustly blame the cold they caught last Campn. it's to be wished our Young Gentlemen would take to some wholesome exercise in Garrison, riding the great horse would be of great service, fencing, playing at tennise, &c: that of doing Garrison duty is a meer triffle & scarcely deserves the name of exercise[c].

[*margin:* Manner of living in Garrison] Their common way of life is making a visite or two in the fore noon, & that in a coach; dressing, & sitting down to dinner at two, & there continue till four or five in the evening, then take coach to the Coffee-house; drinke Coffee or tea, playing Billiards, Draughts, or Bagamonde. tho this be

---

400 Celsus de Medicina, 2.6.17–18. This passage is also quoted by Johnstone, *Historical Dissertation*, p. 28n.

401 Tissot reports (*Essay on Bilious Fevers*, pp. 109–10) that the young patient, a soldier, experienced severe pain for several days, but that it ceased, causing attending practitioners to conclude that gangrene had set in; delirium and lethargy followed, and death shortly afterwards.

334.

[a] **{"Then I go off to sleep, untroubled with the thought that I must rise early on the morrow."}**

Hor: Sat:6. lib:i. V:19.[402]

[b]Dissertation on the Olympic Games by G: West Esq.[403] Alexander broke his horse Bucephalus. See Cyrus's love of hunting, in Xenophon's Cyropaedia.[404] Henry the 4th of France was fond of horses & Dogs. so was King Wm of hunting & horse racing &c.

335. [*continuing on from p. 333*]:

a large Roome, the air is unwholesome from a desagreable heat from a Stove in which sea coale is burnt; all complain of this, especially Phthisicale constitutions, yet cannot refraine going to it, & from hence retire amongst themselves or go to the Tavern, or Playhouse &c: going to the course in fine weather is a favorite diversion, all sit in coaches, bowing to each other en passant, & with some this is the only exercise; few care to get a horseback or ride out for pleasure. many are fond of Concerts, Masquerades, Balls, dress &c:

> **{"Unduly busy in keeping their skins sleek, whose pride it was to sleep till midday and to lull care to rest with the sound of the cithern."}**
>
> Hor: Ep:ii. lb:i.[405]
>
> **{"[The Greeks'] joy was now in flautists, and now in actors of tragedy."}**
>
> Ib: Ep:ii: lb:ii. V.98.[406]
>
> **{"But nowadays all the pleasure even of the knights has passed from the ear to the vain delights of the wandering eye."}**
>
> Ib:[407]
>
> **{"The fight brings danger; while the zither, and night, and Venus, bring delight. Safer is it to lie on the couch, to**

---

[402] Horace, Satires, 1.6.119–20.

[403] Gilbert West, *Odes of Pindar, With Several other Pieces in Prose and Verse, translated from the Greek. To which is Prefixed a Dissertation on the Olympic Games* (London: R. Dodsley, 1749). West does not mention Bucephalus, but Buchanan would in any case not have required a source to note the well-known story of how Alexander broke the horse.

[404] The *Cyropaedia* provides several references to Cyrus as a hunter, esp. 1.4.5–15; Xenophon, *Cyropaedia*, trans. Walter Miller, The Loeb Classical Library (London: William Heinemann; New York: The Macmillan Co., 1914), I, 48–59. According to Xenophon, Cyrus also encouraged boys to spend long hours hunting, in order to toughen themselves physically and mentally: ibid., 1.2.9–11 (Rolfe ed., I, 16–21).

[405] Horace, Epistles, 1.2.29–31.

[406] Ibid., 2.1.98.

[407] Ibid., 2.1.187–8.

clasp a sweetheart in your arms, to tinkle with you fingers the Thracian lyre, than to take in hand the shield, and the spear with sharpened point, and to sustain upon your locks the helmet's weight."}

Ov: Ep:3. V:116.[408]

{"Away from me with your young men arrayed like women!"}

Ib: Ep.4. V.75.[409]

{"Let others go to the wars; let Protesilaus love!"}

Ov: Ep.13. V.84[a].[410]

how much does this differ from Scipio's behaviour in winter quarters when only twenty seven years of age. *et juvenis, et Caelebs, et victor*.[411] says Rollin, he passes the winter, not in idleness & inactivity, not in eating, drinking, & gaming, but to inform himself secretly

336. [*facing p. 335; blank*]

337. [*continuing on from p. 335*]:
of all that related to the enterprize he meditated, & without noise to prepare all that he could to the success of it.[412] when he had taken Carthagena & continued there in garrison he dayly exercised his troops by Sea & land, by which he enured both their bodies & minds to reale battles, by which the Romans were rendered indefatigable, & accustomed to observe in all times & places, the military discipline with the outmost exactness[a].[413]

{"Capua was even then a far from wholesome place for military discipline, and with its means for gratifying every pleasure proved so fascinating to the soldiers that they forgot their native land."} Liv: lb:7.[414]

[*margin:* Deseases in Cantoonment near Antwerp.] Octr.26. N:S: 1745. we cantooned in the neighbourhood of Antwerp; the Officers in good Chateaux, which have been <un>inhabited sometime & are unfurnished, (expecting the army to march this way) are motted round with water & consequently are damp; it's therefore necessary to keep good fires, which all do; the men are quartered with the Peasants, have

408 Ovid, Heroides, 3.116–20.

409 Ibid., 4.75.

410 Ibid., 13.84.

411 "Young, unmarried, and victorious": *Roman History*, V, 359.

412 Ibid., 358; "he passes … success of it" is quoted.

413 Ibid., 360; "enured … exactness" is quoted.

414 Livy, 7.38.5.

good beds, & plenty of fire. the first complaints were sore throats from catching cold at night: it was our custome to pass the evening by visiting at our Country Seats[a.], returning home late, in a thick fog, which is naturale to this Country; many were fond of fishing or sailing in the Motte, & often got cold, bleeding & keeping warm proved a certain cure; the Regmt continued healthie, slight feverish complaints from colds were the only complaints. Genll. Honeywoods Regiment came from Camp directly viz: their quarters in Garrison at Antwerp, & were more sickly

338.

[a.]on his arrival in Africa his first care was to re-establish discipline amongst the troops, which he found entirely ruined. they had neither order, subordination, nor obedience. their sole care was to plunder, eat, drink & divert themselves. he made all the useless mouths quit the camp, regulated the Species of provisions the Sutlers were to bring in, & would suffer none but what were Simple & military, industriously banishing all that tended to luxury & voluptuousness. which cost him neither much time nor pains because he set others the example in his own person. Roll: Rom: hist: Vol:8.[415]

[a.][*sic*] {**"Often a change is pleasant to the rich, and a simple meal beneath the poor man's humble roof, without tapestries and purple, has smoothed the wrinkles on the care-worn brow."**}

Hor: Od:29. lib:3tis.[416]

{**"Visiting the stage oftener than the camp."**}

Justin: lb:vi.[417]

339. [*continuing on from p. 337*]:

than we in our Country quarters; our men lived sober & boarded with their Landlords, which prevented debauches. So soon as our Barracks were prepared for us, we marched into Garrison; the jaundice soon appeared, & some slight fevers from private debauches. the weather was frosty & cold, we had many coughs with pleuretick stiches. We were only a few weeks in Garrison when we were ordered for England; such men as were sicke were greatly concerned in mind, for fear of being left behind in the hospital; which is always the case with Soldiers, none caring to leave their Regmt even when marching to attacke the Enemy. When we marched to relieve Tournay, some sick and lame were carried in waggons, upon hearing an alarm of engaging the Enemy, many quitted the waggons & mounted their horses[a].

---

415 VIII, 195; "first care … own person" is quoted.

416 Horace, Odes, 3.29.13–16.

417 Justin, Trogus, 6.9.4.

{"There is a certain keenness of spirit and impetuosity implanted by nature in all men which is kindled by the ardour of battle. This feeling it is the duty of commanders not to repress but to foster."} Jul: Caesar.[418]

{"There is a division of duties between soldiers and generals; to soldiers belongs the eager enthusiasm for battle, but generals must help by foresight, by counsel, and more often by delay than by rash action."} Tac. Hist: lib:3. cap.20.[419]

{"Yours be the arms and spirit; leave to me the plan of campaign and the direction of your valour."} ib: lib:i. cap.84.[420]

When the mind is so greatly concerned, the body is soon affected, grows restless & unease, tossing & tumbling in bed, nor have medecines the same effect[x], <[x]Pechlin: obs: Med: lib.3. No.13.[421]>, whether given internally or applyed externally, nor do wounds suppurate so kindly in this condition[b].

340.

[a] **{"They await the signal, while throbbing fear and eager passion for glory drain each bounding heart."}**

Virg: Aen:5. V.137.[422]

[*penciled line beside this in right margin*]

[b]I remember Blackburn of Captn Madan's troop ill of the smallpox & likely to do well, yet dyed suddenly on the 9th day. As the troop marched out of town that morning, hearing the Trumpet sound as they pased his window, was greatly concerned, immediately changed, the pustules flattned, his skine became of a deep scarlet colour, fell into violent ravings & dyed that night; the body soon swelled strong & was buried in 24 hours. Bellamy his Comrade was ill at the same time & dyed in the same manner.

341. [*continuing on from p. 339*]:

{"He who fears lest she be his no more, lest someone take her from him, will scarce be healed by Machaon's art [i.e., medicine]."}

---

418 Caesar, Civil Wars, 3.92.

419 Tacitus, Histories, 3.20.

420 Ibid., 1.84.

421 *Observationum*, III, no. 13, pp. 420–2, is entitled, "Imaginationis vires in determinandis medicaminum effectibus" ("The imagination of men in determining the effects of drugs"). Pechlin asserts that the patient's imagination can enhance, diminish, or otherwise alter the effectiveness of drugs in his case.

422 Virgil, Aeneid, 5.137–8.

Ov: rem:Am: V:545.[423]

{"How small a thing, ye mighty gods, to show mercy to one on the eve of death so that at least I might have been covered with my native soil!"}

Ov: trist: lib:3. V:142.[424]

{"So far away, then, on a strange shore I shall die, and the very place shall render harsh my fate."}

Ib. V:149. &c.[425]

Decr. 22d. 1745. we marched out of Garrison for Williamstadt, & such men as were unfit for marching were sent to the hospital yesterday; & three dyed last night unexpectedly, all being greatly concerned at the thoughts of being left behind, & telling their Comrades they should certainly dye. all earnestly wished to return home, yet many dyed.

{"Who seeks his fatherland finds death."} Ramaz: de morb: Artif. C:42.[426]

[*margin:* Deseases in our Dutch Cantoonment.] Decr. 25. we halted at Etten & cantooned amongst the Dutch Booers, the frost preventing our embarking at Wmstadt: many of the men lay upon Straw in barns & outhouses, & tho the weather was cold, they bore it with great patience in hopes of seeing old England soon; Officers were billeted in <the> best houses, & contented, tho badly lodged; all were remarkably healthie, much more so than in Garrison, few complaining of catching cold; they were much in the open air, little or no Duty, & free form town debauches. many <private men> board with their Landlords for Seven Stivers pr day, beer included, live moderately & are sober. all the dirty fellow have the Itch, & say, they catch it from the Boores, who live much on salt pork, hung

342. [*facing p. 341; blank*]

343. [*continuing on from p. 341*]:
beef, Potatoes, &c: We had many scalded feet & toes from sitting near the harth & not accustomed to the heat of turff ashes. Thornton of Captn. Loyd's was slightly scalded on the inside of the right leg, & so much dejected as to take to bed & laye so long in the same posture that the outside of that anckle mortified, attended with slowe fever & dyed. from the first day he was greatly concerned & affraid of the Regmt's marching & leaving him behind them. our Cantoonment is pretty wyde & the sicke in some cases are neglected both as to medecine and nursing; nor do the

---

423 Ovid, Cure for Love, v.545–6.

424 Ovid, Tristia, 3.3.31–2.

425 Ibid., 3.3.37–8.

426 Ramazzini calls this "a camp proverb"; *De morbis artificum* (trans. Wright), p. 369.

men incline to complaine, hoping to get aboard soon & recover at Sea from Seasickness. The Officers were healthie, tho their rooms are cold & smokie, either door or window must be open, yet none complaine. are much abroad, taking country diversions, as skating, shooting, & live soberly. we had some accidents from shooting, by the piece bursting in the hand, & Cornet Frankland's servant lost his hand. our horses improved dayly, being fed at large, not confined to weight, & the hay remarkably good.

[*margin:* Reparations for embarking our horses.] so soon as the frost broke we were ordered to prepare for embarking. as our horses were in good order, bleeding was thought absolutely necessary. some bleed the whole troop, taking three pints from the fattest horses & a quart from the others; but this depends more on the opinion of the Officer than judgement of the Farrier, who is for bleeding the fattest only, thinking it needless to bleed the others on account of the cold weather; tho all were blooded at

344. [*facing p. 343; blank*]

345. [*continuing on from p. 343*]:
our coming over.

[*margin:* Embark at Williamstadt.] Febry. 22nd. N:S: we had a long & dirty march to Wmstadt & embarked that evening, had scarcely time to clean our horses.

> **{"O ye brave heroes, who with me have often suffered worse misfortunes, now banish care with wine! To-morrow we will take again our course over the mighty main."}**
>
> Hor.[427]

the men had the same allowance as in Par:1. the weather being cold we had no occasion to open the Port-holes to air & cool the horses. in small & narrow ships, after being some days aboard, they began to be hot & sweat; it was then necessary to open the Port holes & remove the boat off the hatch-way^{x}.

The men were healthy, only some slight pleureticks & Rheumaticks; bleeding the chief remedy, small punch with Sal: Prunel: their universal drink. after some days it began to be hot & suffocating twixt-decks, & the men were more subject to catch cold when upon decke, few incline to take medecines, expecting to find an infallible cure from Seasickness. when we sailed all were seasicke, as also the greatest part of the Sailors, which they imputed to their lying six weeks in fresh water & within Land; lying quiet & still is reckoned the best preservative against this disorder. Some drink thine chicken or mutton broth in order to

[427] Horace, Odes, 1.7.30–32.

promote vomiting with the greater ease. One of our women was delivered of a child the night before we sailed, having violent grinding pains, I ordered a mixture with a large quantity of Laudanum, of which she took frequently, & was not in the least

346.

in 1625 a grand supply was sent from England, but, by ill management, the forces were kept so long on board the Transports, that an Epidemick distemper broke out amongst them, which differed very little from the Plague, & carried off the greatest part. Biograph: Britannic: V.3. p.1679. Art. Devereux Earl of Essex.[428]

347. [*continuing from p. 345*]:
Sicke during the passage, tho it blew a hard gale & run a very rough sea. our men lived mostly on fresh provisions, which they dayly bought ashore, whilst we remained wind bound at Helvoetslys.

[*margin:* Desembarke at Gravesend.] March 2nd. O:S: 1746: we arrived at Gravesend in high Spirits & well pleased with seeing old England[.]

> **{"... when far off we see dim hills and low-lying Italy. 'Italy!' first Achates shouts aloud; Italy the crews hail with joyful cry."}**
>
> Virg: Aen:3. V:222.[429]

& desembarke our horses in good condition, having lost Six by accidents whilst aboard. as it blew hard during our passage, & tho we were but one night at Sea, many were sick at landing, but soon recovered and fed as usuale. when landed could scarcely walk, their legs being numb'd & stiff, but recovered by gentle exercise and rubbing. some troops were twenty two days on board.

Many men had sore shins from hurts a shipboard as in Par:1. were much inflammed from being so long aboard & wanting poultices; as sea bisket was their only bread, they could not make poultices of the Crumbs, therefore the Meals ought to be kept in readiness. washing with warm water & brandy was their common fomentation, rubbing with brandy was their universal medecine, to which a small quantity of oyle should always be added, otherwise the rag dries too soon & sits into the

348. [*facing p. 347; blank*]

349. [*continuing on from p. 347*]:

---

[428] This passage is actually a quotation: "in 1625 ... greatest part"; *Biog. Brit.*, III, 1679.

[429] Virgil, Aeneid, 3.522–4.

sore. Ungt. Dealth: much used in rubbing the sore parts. Many were itchy, as they lye amongst the dirty hay, & seldom shift nor wash & keep clean. nixt day marched for Country quarters.

{"I have finished my task; hang garlands on the weary vessel; the haven whither my course was set is reached."}

Ov: rem: Amor: V:8ii.[430]

Finis

Authors on Military Diseases & Gunshot Wounds.

A.

ABeille, Le Parfait Chirurgien d'Armee, et Traite de Playes d'Arquebuscade. 8°. Par:1696.

Atkins[.] Navy Surgeon – 1737. 8°.

B.

Brand. (Paul) de Dysenteria Castrensi. extact: Act: Haf: Vol:5. No.3i.
Boscus[.] de Vulneribus a bellico fulmine illatis[.] Ferrariae. 1603. 4to.
Botallus (Leonh) de Sclopitorum Vulneribus. Ven: 1566 & 1598 – 8° – Francf.1575. 4to. Ludg: 1560. 12mo.
Brocklesby (Dr.) Oeconomical & Medical observations. Physician to the Army in Germany. Lon. 1763. 8°.

C.

Chesne (Jos: du) de la Cure des Arquebusades. Lyon 1576. 8°.
Clowes (Wm)[.] a profitable & necessary book of Observations, for all those who are burned with the flame of Gunpowder &c: 1637. 4to.
Coberi[.] Observationes Medicae Castrensium Hungaricarum. Helms. 1685. 4to.
Crausius[.] de Sclopetorum Vulneribus. Jenae. 1695. 4to.
Cockburn's Sea Diseases. 1736. 8°.

D.

Drari (Henr. Franc: Le) Traite ou reflexions sur les playes d'Armes a feu[.] Par: 1737. 8o.
Daillaeus (Peter) de vulneribus ab armis igni vomis inflictis. Par:1668. 12mo.
Traite des Playes d'Armes a feu, par M. Desprot. 12°. 1758.

E.

[430] Ovid, Cure for Love, v.811–2.

F.

Ferrius (Alfonsus) de Sclopetorum Vulneribus[.] Rom. 1552. 4to.
Finckenau (Jac) de Vulneribus Sclopetorum. Regiom: 1716. 4to.
Fonseca (Ant) de Epidemia febrili grassante in exercitu Regis Catholici in inferiori Palatino[.] Anno 1620. & 1621. Mechlinae 1623. 4to.

G:

Gehema (Jani Abrah: a) Medicus et Chirurgus Castrensis[.] Hamb: 1684. 12mo. Germaniae.
Idem – Miles Agrotans. Ibid: 1690. Germaniae.
Gerssorff (Hans Von) Chirurgia Castrensis Argent: 1527. 4to. Germaniae.
Gendre (Ant) de febre Epidemica in Montis Albani obsidione grassata[.] Lugd. 1626. 8o.
Geach (Francis) obs: on inflammations of the eyes, Ulcers, & Gunshot wounds. 1766. 1st.

H:

Heisterus (Laur) de vulneribus Machinarum ignivomarum. Helmst: 1744. 4to.
Hildanus (Fabr: Guil) de partu Caesareo et Vulnere Sclopeti. Oppenh: 1614.
Idem. Cista Militaris[.] Basil: 1633. 8o.
Idem, Nova Chirurgia Castrensis, et Armamentarium Castrense; in quo praecipiae de Gangraena et Sphacelo, de Vulneribus Sclopetorum, Angina et Dysenteria agitur. Basil: 1615. Germaniae.
Hoffmanni (Fred:) Diss: de Militum valetudine tuenda in Castris. Op. Med: Tom:3. p.296. Ed: Genev: – fol. 6. Tom.

I.

K:

Kupferschmidt (Jo) de morbis Praeliantium, quos in victoriosa Bernatum Expeditione bellica 1712 observare Cicuit. Basil. 1715. 4to.

L:

Lebfelter (Jac) de Vulneribus, quae sclopetorum globulis inflicti solent, eorumque Curatione[.] Lips: 1596. 4to.

M:

Maggius (Barthol) de vulnerum Sclopetorum et Bombardarum curatione. Bonon. 1552. 8o.
Idem, de Vulneribus Sclopetorum fol: in Gesneri Scriptoribus optimis chirurgicis. Figur. 1553.
Mindererus (Raymond) Medicina Militaris cum Notis Cardilucci. Norimb: 12. 1679. Germaniae.

Mye (Franc: Vander)de Officio Medici praesidii, et morbis ab urbe recuperata grassantibus Bredanis, erronibus variis Practicorum et medicamentis tempore obsidionis in praesidio pro Militibus praescriptis. Bredae: 1630. 4$^{to.}$
Moyle's Sea Surgeon. 1693. 8$^{o.}$
La Medecine de l'armee. par M: de Meysery. Par. 1754. <3 vol. 12°>.
Monro (Donald) deseases in the British hospital. Lond 1764[.] 8$^{o.}$

N.

O.

P.

Paracelses (Th) Traite des Arquebusades. Lyon. 1581. 8$^{o.}$
Pechlinus (Jo: Nic) de vulneribus Sclopetorum. Kiloni 4to. 1618.
Plazzonus (Franc) de vulneribus Sclopetorum. Ven. 1618. 4$^{to.}$
Portius (Luc: Ant) de Militis in Castris Sanitate tuenda[.] Neap: 1728. 8°.
Pringle's Observations on the Diseases of the Army. Lond: 1752. 8$^{o.}$
Purmannus (Math: Godofr) de vulneribus Sclopetorum. Franc: 1703. 8$^{o.}$ Germaniae.

Q.

Quercetanus (Joseph) de vulneribus Sclopetorum[.] Lugd: 1576. 8$^{o.}$

R:

Ranby on Gunshot Wounds. Lond: 1743. 8$^{o.}$
Romanus (Franc) de militari Medicinae conditione[.] Neap.
Rota (Jo: Franc) de Tormentiorum vulnerum natura et Conditione[.] Bonon: 1555. 4to.
Idem, de Sclopetorum vulneribus. Ven:1566. 8$^{o.}$
Rouppe (Ludovic:) M. D: de morbis Navigantis. L.B. 1764. 8$^{o.}$

S.

Sartorius (Joh: Geo) de morbo militari, seu Castrensi, Bambergae. 1684. fol:
Sancassani (Diomisii Andre) Chirurgie Castrensis. 8$^{o.}$ Ven. 1708. Italiae.
Schmidii (Andr. Chr.) Chirurgia Militaris Franc: 12to. 1664. Germaniae.
Snebergerus (Ant) de bona militum valetudine conservanda Cracoviae 1564. 8$^{o.}$

T.

Tassins (Leonh) Chirurgie ou L'Art de querir les playes d'Arquebusades. Par: 1683. 8$^{o.}$

W.

Willius (Joh: Valent) de morbis Castrensibus internis. Hafnie. 1676. 4$^{to.}$
Verbrugs (Jo:) Chirurgia terretris et Navalis. 8$^{o.}$ Amst. 1704. Belgiae.
Van Swieten. Maladies de l'armee. Par. 8$^{o.}$ 1761.

X

Y.

Z.

Zwingerus (Theodor) de morbis Praeliantium[.] Basil: 1715. 4to.

[*inserted sheets, #1*]

[*inserted sheets, #2*]

[*beginning of fragment*] -ous in eating fruite especially such as are naturally dispos'd to this distemper; as also not to be affraid of catching the distemper vid: p. 60.[431] says the chief cause of it is within ourselves p.61. but so subtile if it escapes our Senses, in the beginning theres something Acrid, caustic, & corrosive, which irritates the Stomach & Guts; after endevouring to explain it in a more easie & plain manner, than has been customary with Physicians, & attempting to avoid cramp words, at last ends in saying it was of an Arsenick quality vid p.77, 81. his method of cure was universally the same in both Sexes, all Ages & constitutions, VIZ: beginning with a vomite of Ipecacoan, tho in many cases this was not absolutely necessary therefor gave the Rhabarb immede<a>tely & repeated it at any time of the desease. did not use it so much in powder as in tincture prepar'd according to Rofinus method. {**Take ½ oz. rhubarb, 1 dr. salt of tartar, mentholated chicory water ...**} or any other distill'd water, oz.v or vi. ordering a Spoonfull every four or Sixe hours according to the Constitution vid. 107. on this he depended & it seldom fail'd; if the flux continued cort: Simarube dr.ii. was boyled in {**a quantity of water sufficient to leave, when boiled, 8 oz.[of decoction]**} drinking oz.i or ii. every 3 or 4 hours till well 115. if the desease withstood the above method, continuing from a lax habit of body, then he us'd gentle astringents viz: Cort: Cascarillae & Suc: Catechu. such as had violent griepings he gave sweet oyle as much as the Patient could take, dissolving Gum Arabic or Tragacanth in Decoct: Simarubae; giving clysters ex ol: Lin: which he prefers to all other oyles. Suspects Opiates saying they ought to be given with great caution. in case

---

[431] In the chapter to which Buchanan is referring here, Degner reviews various common opinions on what causes dysentery. He generally argues against the assertions, including (*Historia medica*, pp. 57–60) the one that fruit is to blame.

of Strangury a few drops Bals: Sulphur prov'd a cure. feverish complaints were taken off with gentle Diaphoreticks & Absorbents. theriac plaister or e crusta pan: alb Vino rubio & Nuce Moschata being applyed to the belly asswaged pains. recommends an antialcalescent Dyet viz. Barley, Rice, Panada &c with milk, forbidding every thing that's acide or of bad digestion. Drink of the same natures sharpned with juice of Lemons which was very serviceable in this desease, as was also butter milk. recommends Rhenish & Mosell wines, claret not so proper. if it continued obstinate strengtheners must be used, for this purpose was his Tinct. tonica. {**Take tincture of antimony with prepared spirit of hartshorn, tincture of vitriol, and *Martis Ludovicus*, small quantities of each**} care being taken sometime afterwards of a proper Regimen. having deliver'd his own method of cure, he then gives a large acct. of what methods are used by private families & Quacks, & his opinion of them amounting to 34. afterwards treats of a preservative method to avoid this desease; saying that the same medecines wch cure a desease will likewise preserve us from it, if prudently manag'd, therefor a Spoonfull or two of the Rhabarb tincture should be taken every morning, or its powder, 1st giving the Ipecacoan if necessary. the Dyet of easie Digestion sharpen'd with Vinegar & juice of Lemons, to drink Rhenish or Mosell wine, a moderate use of fruit may be serviceable by keeping the body open p. 165. recommends cleanleness; necessary houses should be appointed purposely for the deseased, no communication to be kep't with them. then mentions the vulgar method us'd to prevent it. afterwards has some particular observations & cautions on the method of treating this desease, saying that bleeding was seldome usefull rather prejudiciale; astringents seldom necessary; reckons Rhab: the universal remedy, honouring it with the title of Divine medecine & should never be wasted, the whole is very distinct & told in a plain short manner with great appearance of truth, giving an instance or two of his general method of practice, had pag. 200 L.P: with a good Index. To this is added a very particular Case of the bad effects of Mercur: Sublim: corrosiv: applyed in a plaister to a small Tumor on the Thigh of a Lady aged fourty Seven years of a good constitution; guesses this might be three half Scruples in the whole, tho applyed at three different times, occasion'd a very large & thick Eschar, a violent Salivation & all the bad Symptoms that could possibly attend it, for wch it was no remedy, the very bones being affected with foetid ulcers. this was practic'd by an itinerant Quack, the case being so remarkable was laid befor the Magistrates. the Quack endeavour'd to vindicate himself wch he Supports with nine Arguments, the case is afterwards refer'd to the faculty of Physicians & You have their answer condemning the practice. This is well told in a plain easie Style, as also his method of practice he attempted to save the Patient's life; in the Epistle to the Reader, he is very severe on all Quacks, to them he joins

Camp-Surgeons, saying their Education is at first in the barbar's Shop, then learning to bleed & dress slight wounds, & from being attendants at chirurgical operations, become profess'd Surgeons & are appointed as such to some troop or Company, where they practice at random & learn a particular method. afterwards assume the name of Doctors[.] this may probably be true in his Country, & is customary in Germany & the Low Countries, all Barbars practising Surgery, commonly illiterate, tho some are smatterers in Latin, entirely ignorant of Anatomy, few or none having ever seen a Desection, nor is the profession much esteem'd. they have hardly a book, nor do they knowe any. Our Regimtal Surgeons from the beginning are generally well educated; wheither they are to profess Physick or Surgery have the same education, first serving an apprenticeship are instructed in all the particular branches of medecine & Surgery by proper Professors, attending the Lectures two or three years; & for further improvement travele to forreing [*sic*] universities & attend hospitals, of wch Paris & Leiden have been the most remarkable; some go to Montpellier making the tour of Italy, afterwards many take to the army in order to pass some years, & there officiate as Physician, Surgeon & Apothecary; tho young Practitioners are sure of practice & may improve by experience; supposing equal capacities the advantage most [*sic*] be very considerable.

The Author charges <us> with using dangerous & poysenous medecines, Such as Mercur: Sublim: corrosiv: & that without weight or measure, & says it's our common practice to give Arsenick inwardly in order to cure intermittent fevers. I'm intimately acquainted with the greatest part of the Regimental Surgeons of our Army, & can positively affirm that no such medecines are used by them; We have a weekly Club w<h>ere all are welcome to come, the chief Subject of conversation relates to our own business; it being a standing rule with us, that if any thing remarkable happen'd during the last weeks practice, it's to be made publick for the good of the Society; by this means we know the practice of the whole army during the Campn, & in winter quarters that of the Garrison, where we have an opportunity of attending the hospital. All talk freely, nor can I perceive any reservedness or fondness for Secret medecines, or a private method of practice; some are regular bred Physicians. I take the practice of the whole to be fair & honest, free from the superfluity of pompous [*end of fragment*]

Bibliography

Manuscript Sources

British Library:
  Additional 6861 (Pringle-Mitchell correspondence)
Church of Jesus Christ of Latter-Day Saints:
  International Genealogical Index
Guildhall Library, London:
  Records of the Society of Apothecaries, Freedom Books
National Archives (formerly, the Public Record Office), London:
  Probate 11
  State Papers 41
  War Office 27
  War Office 64
National Army Museum, London:
  Cumberland's orderly book, Dec. 1745–June 1747
Staffordshire Records Office, Stafford:
  D685 (Records of Stafford General Infirmary)
  Parish Register for St Mary's, Births and Burials 1760–1801
  Parish Register for St Mary's, Marriages 1754–1787
Wellcome Library for the History & Understanding of Medicine, London
  John Hawkins journal (Ms. 2788)
  John Buchanan, "Regimental Practice. or A Short History of Diseases common to His Majesties own Royal Regiment of Horse Guards when abroad (Commonly called the Blews)" (RAMC 1037)
Windsor Castle
  Cumberland Papers

Classical Works

Celsus. *De Medicina*, trans. W.G. Spencer. The Loeb Classical Library (Cambridge, Mass.: Harvard Univ. Press; London: William Heinemann Ltd, 1960 [1935]. 3 vols.

Dioscorides. *The Greek Herbal of Dioscorides*, trans. John Goodyer, ed. Robert T. Gunther. Oxford: Oxford Univ. Press, 1934.

Hippocrates. *Hippocrates*. trans. and ed. W.H.S. Jones (vols. 1–2, 4), E.T. Withington (vol. 3) and Paul Potter (vols. 5–6). The Loeb Classical Library. London: William Heinemann, Ltd; New York: G.P. Putnam's Sons, 1923–31;

Cambridge, Mass.: Harvard Univ. Pr.; London: William Heinemann Ltd, 1988. 6 vols.

Horace. *Horace. Satires, Epistles and Ars Poetica.* trans. H. Rushton Fairclough, The Loeb Classical Library. Cambridge, Mass.: Harvard Univ. Press; London: William Heinemann Ltd, 1955 [1926].

Pindar. *Odes of Pindar, With Several other Pieces in Prose and Verse, Translated from the Greek. To which is Prefixed a Dissertation on the Olympic Games.* Trans. and introd. Gilbert West. London: R. Dodsley, 1749.

Xenophon. *Cyropaedia.* trans. Walter Miller. The Loeb Classical Library. London: William Heinemann; New York: The Macmillan Co., 1914. 2 vols.

Works Published 1500–1820, Relating to Medicine, Surgery, and Pharmaceuticals

Abercromby, David. *De variatone, ac varietate pulsus observationes.* London: Samuelis Smith, 1685.

Baglivi, Giorgio. *De praxi medica ad priscam observandi rationem revocanda. Libri duo. Accedunt dissertationes novae.* Leiden: Fredericum Haring, 1704.

——. *The Practice of Physick, Reduc'd to the Ancient Way of Observations. Containing a Just Parallel between The Wisdom and Experience of the Ancients, and The Hypothesis's of Modern Physicians. Intermixed With many Practical Remarks upon most Distempers.* London: Andrew Bell [etc.], 1704.

Ball, John. *The Modern Practice of Physic: or a Method of judiciously Treating the Several Disorders incident to the Human Body.* London: A. Millar, 1760. 2 vols.

Barker, John. *An Essay on the Agreement betwixt Ancient and Modern Physicians: Or a Comparison Between the Practice of Hippocrates, Galen, /Sydenham, and Boerhaave, in Acute Diseases. Intended to Shew, What the Practice of Physick, in such Distempers, ought to be.* London: G. Hawkins, 1747.

Boerhaave, Herman. *Boerhaave's Aphorisms: Concerning the Knowledge and Cure of Diseases.* 3rd ed. London: W. Innys [etc.], 1755.

Brocklesby, Richard. *Oeconomical and Medical Observations, In Two Parts, From the Year 1758 to the Year 1763, inclusive: Tending to The Improvement of Military Hospitals, and to The Cure of Camp Diseases incident to Soldiers.* London: T. Becket and P.A. De Hondt, 1764.

Carr, Richard. *Dr. Carr's Medicinal Epistles Upon Several Occasions: Done into English, as a Supplement to the Explanations of Sanctorious's Aphorisms,* trans. John Quincy. London: William Newton and J. Phillips, 1714.

——. *Epistolae medicinales variis occasionibus conscriptae.* London: Stafford Anson, 1691.

Castro, Rodrigo de. *Medicus-politicus: sive, De officiis medico-politicis tractatus, quatuor distinctus libris: in quibus non solum bonorum medicorum mores ac virtutes exprimuntur, malorum vero fraudes & imposturae deteguntur, verum etiam pleraque, alia circa novum hoc argumentum utilia atque iucunda exactissime proponuntur*. Hamburg: Bibliopolio Frobeniano, 1614.

Champney, Thomas. *Medical and Chirurgical Reform Proposed, from a Review of the Healing Art, throughout Europe, particularly Great Britain*. London: J. Johnson [etc.], 1797.

Dancer, Thomas. *A Brief History of the Recent Expedition against Fort San Juan, So far as it Relates to the Diseases of the Troops; together with Some Observations on Climate, Infection and Contagion; and Several of the Endemial Complaints of the West-Indies*. Kingston: D. Douglas & W. Aikman, 1781.

Degner, Johann Hartmann. *Historia medica de dysenteria bilioso-contagiosa*. Utrecht, 1738.

Diemerbroeck, Ysbrand van. *Tractatus copiosissimus de peste*. Geneva, 1721. 2 vols.

Dunne, Charles. *The Chirurgical Candidate; or, Reflections on Education: Indispensable to Complete Naval, Military, and Other Surgeons*. London: Samuel Highley, 1808.

"E. R." *The Experience'd Farrier: Or, a Compleat Treatise of Horsemanship. In Two Books; Physical and Chyrurgical*. 2nd ed., enl. London: W. Whitwood and A. Feltham, 1691.

Hamilton, Robert. *The Duties of a Regimental Surgeon Considered: With Observations on His General Qualifications; And Hints relative to a More Respectable Practice, and Better Regulation of that Department*. London, J. Johnson [etc.], 1787. 2 vols.

Heister, Laurence. Medical, *Chirurgical, and Anatomical Cases and Observations*. trans. George Wirgman. London: J. Reeves [etc.], 1755.

Hoffman, Friedrich. *Opera omnia physico-medica denuò revisa, correcta & aucta, in sex tomos distributa*. Geneva: fratres de Tournes, 1740. 6 vols. In 3.

——. *A System of the Practice of Medicine: From the Latin of Dr. Hoffman*. trans. William Lewis, rev. Andrew Duncan. London: J. Murray, 1783. 2 vols.

Home, Francis. *Medical Facts and Experiments*. London: A. Millar; Edinburgh: A. Kincaid and J. Bell, 1759.

Huxham, John. *An Essay on Fevers*. Introd. Saul Jarcho. Canton, Mass.: Science History Publications [Eatson Publishing Intl.], 1988; repr. of 3rd [1757] ed.

——. *Observationes de aere et morbis epidemicis, ab anno M DCC XXVIII ad finem anni M DCC XXXVII*, London: Joannes Hinton [etc.],1739–52. 2 vols.

——. *Observations on the Air and Epidemic Diseases From the Year MDCCXXVIII to MDCCXXXVII. inclusive; Made by Dr. Huxham, at Plymouth: Together with a Short Dissertation on the Devonshire Colic. Translated from the Latin Original, and now Published with the Doctor's Approbation*. London: J. Hinton and Henry Whitfeld, 1759–67. 2 vols.

James, Robert. *A Medicinal Dictionary; Including Physic, Surgery, Anatomy, Chymistry, and Botany. In all their Branches relative to Medicine. Together with a History of Drugs; An Account of thir Various Preparations, Combinations, and Uses; And An Introductory Preface, tracing the Progress of Physic, and explaining the Theories which have principally prevail'd in all Ages of the World*. London: T. Osborne, 1743–45. 3 vols.

Johnstone, James. *An historical dissertation concerning the malignant epidemical fever of 1756*. London, 1758.

Le Pois, Charles. *Selectiorum observationum et consiliorum*. noviss. ed. Leiden: Cornelii Boutestein and Joh. Arnoldum, 1714.

The Medical Register For the Year 1783. London: Joseph Johnson, [1783].

Moore, John. *Medical Sketches: In Two Parts*. 1st American ed. Providence, R.I., Carter & Wilkinson, 1794.

Pechlin, Johann Nicolaus. *Observationum physico-medicarum libri tres, quibus accessit, Ephemeris vulveris thoracici & in eam commentarius*. Hamburg: Libraria Schultziana, 1691. 2 vols in 1.

The Practice of the British and French Hospitals: Viz. The Edinburgh, Military, and Naval Hospital, / L'Hotel Dieu, La Charite, and Les Invalides. Containing A select Body of useful and elegant Medicines For the several Disorders incident to the Human Body; with Practical Remarks on each Prescription. 2nd ed. London: R. Baldwin, 1775.

Pringle, John. *Observations on the Diseases of the Army, in Camp and Garrison: In Three Parts: With an Appendix, Containing some Papers of Experiments, Read at several Meetings of the Royal Society*. 2nd ed., corr. and enl. London: A. Millar [etc.], 1753.

Quincy, John *Lexicon Physico-Medicum: Or, A New Physical Dictionary, Explaining The Difficult Terms used in the several Branches of the Profession, and in such Parts of Philosophy as are introductory thereunto. To which is added, Some Account of the Things Signified by such Terms. Collected From the most eminent Authors, and particularly those who have wrote upon Mechanical Principles.* London: Andrew Bell, William Taylor, and John Osborn, 1719.

Ramazzini, Bernardini *De Morbis artificum Bernardini Ramazzini diatriba: Diseases of Workers. The Latin Text of 1713*. trans. and ed. Wilmer Cave Wright. Chicago: Univ. of Chicago P., 1940.

——, and Luigi Cornaro. *L'art de conservar la santé des princes .. et Les avantages de la vie sobre*. Leiden, 1724.

Ranby, John. *The Method of Treating Gunshot Wounds*. 2nd ed. London: Robert Horsfield, 1760.

Reide, Thomas Dickson. *A View of the Diseases of the Army in Great Britain, America, the West Indies, and on Board of King's Ships and Transports, from the Beginning of the Late War to the Present Time. Together with Monthly and Annual Returns of the Sick, and Some Account of the Method in Which They were Treated in the Twenty-Ninth Regiment, and the Third Battalion of the Sixtieth Regiment.* London: J. Johnson, 1793.

Rollo, John. *Observations on the Diseases which Appeared in the Army on St. Lucia, in December, 1778; January, February, March, April, and May, 1779. To Which are Prefixed, Remarks Calculated to Assist in Ascertaining the Causes, and in Explaining the Treatment, of Those Diseases. With an*

Appendix, Containing a Short Address to Military Gentlemen, on the Means of Preserving Health in the West-Indies. 2nd ed., rev. Barbadoes and London: Charles Dilly, 1781.

Russell, Richard. *Oeconomia naturae in morbis acutis et chronicis glandularum.* London, 1755.

——. *The Oeconomy of Nature in Acute and Chronical Diseases of the Glands.* London: J. and J. Rivington, 1755.

Santorio Santorio [Sanctorius Sanctorius]. *Aphorismi de medicina statica.* Leipzig: Joann. Michael. Ludov. Teubner, 1762.

——. *Medicina Statica: Being the Aphorisms of Sanctorius, Translated into English with large Explanations. Wherein is given A Mechanical Account of the Animal Oeconomy, and of the Efficacy of the Non-Naturals, either in bringing about or removing its Disorders: Also with an Introduction concerning Mechanical Knowledge, and the Grounds of Certainty in Physick.* trans. and ed. John Quincy. London: William Newton, 1712.

Sprengell, [Conrad Joachim]. "Observations on Dr. Eaton's Styptic." *Philosophical Transactions of the Royal Society of London*, 33 (1724–25), pp. 108–14.

Stevenson, William. *Considerations on the Dangerous Effects of Promiscuous Blood-letting.* Newark, 1783.

"Sur la maniere d'arrester les hemorrhages, qui viennent après de membres coupés," *Histoire de l'Académie royale de sciences*, 1733. Paris: Impr. Royale, 1735. pp. 30–32.

Tissot, Samuel. *Essay on Bilious Fevers; or, The History of a Bilious Epidemic Fever at Lausanne, in the Year MDCCLV.* London: D. Wilson and T. Durham, 1760.

Tulp, Nicolaas. *Observationes medicae.* 6th ed. Leiden: Georgium Wishoff, 1739.

Turner, Daniel. *Syphilis: A Practical Dissertation on the Venereal Disease.* 4th ed., rev. London: J. Walthoe [etc.], 1732.

Weber, Philipp. *Thermarum Wisbadensium description. Complectens antiquitatem et utilitatem harum thermarum.* Oppenheim: Hieronymi Galleri, 1617.

Whytt, Robert. *An Essay on the Virtues of Lime-Water in the Cure of the Stone.* Edinburgh: Hamilton, Balfour, and Neill, 1752.

Young, George. *A Treatise on Opium, Founded upon Practical Observations.* London: A. Millar, 1753.

Other Published Primary Sources

Aleyn, Charles. *The Battailes of Crescey and Poictiers: under the Fortunes and Valour of King Edward the Third of that Name, and His Sonne Edward Prince of Wales, Named the Black.* 2nd ed., enl. London: Thomas Knight, 1633.

Anderson, Peter John, comp. *Fasti Academiae Mariscallanae Aberdonensis: Selections from the Records of the Marischal College and University MDXCIII–MDCCCLX.* Aberdeen: New Spalding Club, 1898.

The Army List of 1740. Sheffield: Sir W.C. Ling & Co., Ltd [for the Society for Army Historical Research], 1931.

Army Lists: 1756, 1763, 1767, 1768.

Biographia Britannica: or, The Lives of the Most Eminent Persons Who have Flourished in Great Britain and Ireland, from the Earliest Ages, down to the Present Times. London: W. Innys [etc.], 1747–66. 6 vols. in 7.

Buchanan, George. "George Buchanan's *Elegies* and *Silvae* Translated, with Introduction and Commentary." trans. and ed. David Henry Sabrio, unpub. Ph.D. diss., Univ. of South Carolina, 1980.

Carte, Thomas. *A General History of England*. London: printed for the author, 1747–55. 4 vols.

The City and Court Register: 1744, 1746.

Cooper, John Gilbert. *The Life of Socrates: Collected from the Memorabilia of Xenophon and the Dialogues of Plato*. London: R. Dodsley, 1749.

Gentleman's Magazine: 1749, 1751, 1755, 1767.

Johnston, William, comp. *Roll of Commissioned Officers in the Medical Services of the British Army who Served on Full Pay within the Period between the Accession of George II and the Formation of the Royal Army Medical Corps, 20 June 1727 to 23 June 1898, With an Introduction Showing the Historical Evolution of the Corps*. Harry A.L. Howell, ed. Aberdeen: Aberdeen University Press, 1917. Repr. in A. Peterkin, William Johnston, and Robert Drew, *Commissioned Officers in the Medical Services of the British Army 1660–1960*, vol. I. [Publications of the Wellcome Historical Medical Library, Historical Monograph Series, no. 14.] London: The Wellcome Historical Medical Library, 1968. 2 vols.

Journal of the Campaign on the Coast of France, 1758. London: J. Townsend, 1758.

Leland, Thomas. *The Life and Reign of Philip King of Macedon, the Father of Alexander*. 2nd ed. London: E. Johnston, 1775. 2 vols.

London Magazine. 1751, 1752.

Montaigne, Michel de. *The Essays of Montaigne*. Trans. John Florio, introd. J.I.M. Stewart. New York: The Modern Library, n.d.

Montesquieu, Charles Louis de Secondat, Baron de. *Reflections on the Causes of the Rise and Fall of the Roman Empire*, 2nd ed., enl. London: W. Innys [etc.], 1752. 2 vols.

Parker, Robert. Memoirs of the Most Remarkable Military Transactions from the Year 1683 to 1718. *Containing a Very Particular Account of the Several Battles, Sieges, &c. in Ireland and Flanders during the Reigns of K. William and Q. Anne*. Dublin: Geo. and Alex. Ewing, 1746.

Pereira, Benito. *Commentarium et disputationum in Genesim*. Coloniae Aggripinae, 1601.

Peterkin, Alfred, comp., *A List of Commissioned Medical Officers of the Army: Charles II. to Accession of George II. 1660 to 1727*. Repr. in A. Peterkin, William Johnston, and Robert Drew, *Commissioned Officers in the Medical*

Services of the British Army 1660–1960, vol. I. [Publications of the Wellcome Historical Medical Library, Historical Monograph Series, no. 14.] London: The Wellcome Historical Medical Library, 1968. 2 vols.

Rollin, Charles. *The Roman History from the Foundation of Rome to the Battle of Actium: That is, To the End of the Commonwealth.* rev. ed. Dublin, R. Reilly, 1743. 16 vols.

Sallengre, Albert Henri de. *L'Eloge de L'Yvresse.* La Haye: Pierre Gosse, 1714.

Salmon, Thomas. *The Universal Traveller; or, A complete description of the several nations of the World.* London: R. Baldwin, 1752–53. 2 vols.

Scots Magazine, 1767.

Smollett, Tobias George. *A Complete History of England, from the Descent of Julius Caesar, to the Treaty of Aix-la- Chapelle, 1748.* 2nd ed. London, J. Rivington [etc.], 1758–60. 11 vols.

Thompson, James. *The Seasons.* ed. James Sambrook. Oxford: Oxford Univ. Press, 1981.

Wallis, P.J. and R.V., comps. *Eighteenth-Century Medics (Subscriptions, Licences, Apprenticeships).* 2nd ed. Newcastle-upon-Tyne: Project for Historical Biobibliography, 1988.

Secondary Sources

Arthur, (Sir) George. *The Story of the Household Cavalry.* London: Archibald Constable & Co. Ltd, 1909. 2 vols.

Boog Watson, William N. "Thomas Robertson, Naval Surgeon, 1793–1828." *Bulletin of the History of Medicine*, 46 (1972), pp. 131–49.

Burnby, Juanita G.L. *A Study of the English Apothecary from 1660 to 1760.* [Medical History, supp. no. 3.] London: Wellcome Institute for the History of Medicine, 1983.

Curth, Louise Hill. "The Care of the Brute Beast: Animals and the Seventeenth-century Medical Market-place." *Social History of Medicine*, 15 (2002), pp. 375–92.

Dictionary of National Biography. ed. (Sir) Leslie Stephen and (Sir) Sidney Lee. New York: Macmillan Co.; London: Smith, Elder & Co., 1908–09. 22 vols.

Ditchfield, P.H., and William Page, eds. *The Victoria History of Berkshire.* vol. III. London: St. Catherine Press, 1923.

Fortescue, (Sir) John. W. *A History of the British Army.* 2nd ed. London: Macmillan and Co., Ltd, 1910–30. 13 vols. in 19.

French, Roger K. *Robert Whytt, The Soul, and Medicine.* London: Wellcome Institute, 1969.

Garnier, Arthur E. *The Chronicles of the Garniers of Hampshire during Four Centuries, 1530–1900.* London: Jarrold, 1900.

Gray, Ernest A. "John Hunter and Veterinary Medicine." *Medical History*, 1 (1957), pp. 38–50.

Howell, H.A.L. "The Story of the Army Surgeon and the Care of the Sick and Wounded in the British Army, from 1715 to 1748." *Journal of the Royal Army Medical Corps*, 22 (1914), pp. 320–34, 455–71.

Hume, Edgar Erskine. "Francis Home, M.D. (1719–1813). The Scottish Military Surgeon Who First Described Diphtheria as a Clinical Entity." *Bulletin of the History of Medicine*, 11 (1942), pp. 48–68.

Kopperman, Paul E. "The British Army in North America and the West Indies, 1755–1783: A Medical Perspective." *War, Medicine and Britain, 1600–1800*, ed. Geoffrey Hudson. Amsterdam: Rodopi Press [Clio Medica/Wellcome Historical Institute Series in the History of Medicine], 2007, pp. 51–86.

——. "The British High Command and Soldiers' Wives in America, 1755–1783." *Journal of the Society for Army Historical Research*, 60 (1982), pp. 14–34.

——. "The Drive toward More Moderate Therapies in British Medicine, 1750–1800." *Proceedings of the 37th International Congress on the History of Medicine* (2002), pp. 266–74.

Rolleston, Humphry. "Medical Aphorisms, Chiefly in English." *Bulletin of the History of Medicine*, 10 (1941), pp. 544–67.

Singer, Dorothea Waley. "Sir John Pringle and His Circle." *Annals of Science*, 6 (1949), pp. 127–80.

Stevenson, Lloyd G. "A Note on the Relation of Military Service to Licensing in the History of British Surgery." *Bulletin of the History of Medicine*, 27 (1953), pp. 420–27.

Townshend, C.V.F. *The Military Life of Field-Marshal George First Marquess Townshend 1724–1807*. London: John Murray, 1901.

Williams, Cyril. The *Staffordshire General Infirmary: A History of the Hospital from 1765*. [Stafford:] Mid-Staffordshire General Hospital, 1992.

Index

* 9 7 8 0 7 5 4 6 6 8 7 7 0 *

T - #0010 - 271120 - C0 - 234/156/13 [15] - CB - 9780754668770 - Gloss Lamination